Multiple Sclerosis
in Clinical Practice

Multiple Sclerosis in Clinical Practice

Stanley van den Noort, MD, Professor
Department of Neurology
University of California, Irvine
and
Chief Medical Officer
National Multiple Sclerosis Society

and

Nancy J. Holland, EdD
Vice President, Clinical Programs Department
National Multiple Sclerosis Society

8/2 001

Demos Medical Publishing, Inc., 386 Park Avenue South, New York, New York 10016

Library of Congress Cataloging-in-Publication Data

Available from the publisher upon request

Printed in Canada

Preface

Almost half a million people suffer from and are diagnosed with multiple sclerosis (MS) in North America, and an unknown number suffer from MS and are not yet diagnosed. With this prevalence, most primary care clinicians will have at least one or two patients with MS in their practice.

Although glucocorticoids have long been the mainstay for the symptomatic treatment of acute episodes of MS, only since 1993 have effective treatments, such as beta interferon and glatiramer acetate, been available that alter the course and progression of the disease.

Changes in our ability to diagnose and treat MS have created a paradox, shared with other serious, complicated chronic diseases such as HIV/AIDS. Multiple sclerosis has become at the same time both more of a primary care *and* subspecialty care disease. With more effective treatment options, the complexity of optimal management requires more and more subspecialty expertise, all the while heightening the importance of the primary care clinician's role in early diagnosis and long-term comanagement. The collaboration of the patient, primary care physician, MS specialist, and other members of the health care team (i.e., nurses, physical and occupational therapists, and others) becomes even more essential for optimal care.

As a family physician, I learned four important points from *Multiple Sclerosis in Clinical Practice:*

  1. Effective, disease-modifying treatments are now available, making early diagnosis and initiation of treatment imperative.

2. New diagnostic tools, such as magnetic resonance imaging (MRI), may place the astute primary care physician in the role of making a diagnosis previously made by neurologists who specialize in MS.
3. These more powerful diagnostic methods may shorten the limbo before diagnosis (i.e., "symptoms separated by space and time") but place the acute grief reaction to the diagnosis of a chronic disease with an uncertain prognosis in the primary care physician's office.
4. Patients with MS suffer, of course, from many other common conditions, including pseudoexacerbations.

The legacy of waiting and waiting—sometimes for years—for the disease to manifest itself clearly enough for a definitive diagnosis is now history but means new responsibilities for the primary care physician, both in diagnosis and in long-term comanagement with MS specialists.

My personal experience may not be typical but my professional experience with MS probably is. I have one patient in my practice with MS whose many other problems, including cerebral blindness due to head trauma from domestic violence, dwarf her MS symptoms.

A nurse practitioner colleague has been diagnosed with MS after separate episodes of optic neuritis but has had no further progression. Why I am writing this Foreword comes from more personal experience. My best friend—Patricia Robertson Amusa-Shonubi—died in 1994 from what her neurologist, an MS specialist, described as the worst case of MS he had ever seen. Treatment came too late for Pat, and her primary care was tragic too, but with what you will find in this book, you will be able to ensure that others will not have to suffer her fate.

A. H. Strelnick, M.D.
Professor, Family Medicine
Montefiore Medical Center
Albert Einstein College of Medicine
Bronx, New York

Foreword

Those of us who work with people who have multiple sclerosis (MS) are acutely aware of the enormously difficult consequences of this disease, for both the individuals with MS and their loved ones. We are, however, fortunate to be living in a time more promising than ever before—treatments to alter the disease course and relieve many symptoms are now available. It remains for you, the physician, to bring these therapies to your patients with MS. This is certainly a wonderful opportunity, as well as a difficult challenge, given the complexities and enigma of this difficult disease.

As you provide health care for people with MS, the National Multiple Sclerosis Society is your partner, providing programs to support those with MS, their families, as well as the physicians and allied health professionals. We at the Society thank you for your dedication, knowledge, and skill in assisting people with MS. Together we will advance the mission of the National Multiple Sclerosis Society, "to end the devastating effects of MS."

Gen. Michael J. Dugan, USAF, Ret.
President & CEO
National Multiple Sclerosis Society

Dedication

This book is dedicated to those with multiple sclerosis and to their families. They show great spirit, courage, patience, and optimism. They know that their glasses are half full. May those who read this serve them better.

To Byron Waksman, M.D., the father of modern research in multiple sclerosis.

S. V. D. N.

To my husband, Bill, and daughter, Stephanie, with loving appreciation for your support.

To Labe Scheinberg, M.D., who insisted that people with multiple sclerosis could be helped, then showed a generation of health care professionals how to do it.

N. J. H.

Acknowledgments

The editors wish to thank Dr. Diana Schneider and Joan Wolk for their editorial assistance.

We also acknowledge the ongoing efforts of the National Multiple Sclerosis Society to advance its mission to end the devastating effects of multiple sclerosis by improving quality of care for those with MS through physician education activities.

Contents

Contributors

Timothy L. Vollmer, MD, Director
Yale University Multiple Sclerosis Research Center
40 Temple Street, Suite 71
New Haven, Connecticut

Stanley van den Noort, MD, Professor
Department of Neurology
University of California, Irvine
100 Irvine Hall
Irvine, California
  and
Chief Medical Officer
National Multiple Sclerosis Society
733 Third Avenue
New York, New York

Randall T. Schapiro, MD
The Fairview University Multiple Sclerosis Center
701 25th Avenue South, Suite 200
Minneapolis, Minnesota

Diana M. Schneider, Ph.D., Publisher
Demos Medical Publishing
386 Park Avenue South, Suite 201
New York, New York

Heidi Wynn Maloni, BSN, CNRN
The Catholic University of America
School of Nursing
Washington, DC

Kathleen C. Kobashi, MD
Fellow, Tower Urology Institute for Continence
Cedars-Sinai Medical Center
Los Angeles, California

Gary E. Leach, MD
Director, Tower Urology Institute for Continence
Cedars-Sinai Medical Center
Clinical Professor or Urology, University of Southern California
Los Angeles, California

Nancy J. Holland, EdD
Vice President, Clinical Programs Department
National Multiple Sclerosis Society
New York, New York

Elliot M. Frohman, MD, PhD
Department of Neurology
Director, Multiple Sclerosis Program and Eye Movement Clinics
Southwestern Medical School
5323 Harry Hines Boulevard
Dallas, Texas

Randolph B. Schiffer, MD
The Vernon and Elizabeth Haggerton Chair in Neurology
Department of Neuropsychiatry and Behavioral Science
Texas Tech University Health Sciences Center
Lubbock, Texas

Linda Samuel, MSW
Senior Consultant, Clinical Programs Department
National Multiple Sclerosis Society
733 Third Avenue
New York, New York

Pamela Cavallo, MSW, CSW
Director, Clinical Programs Department
National Multiple Sclerosis Society
733 Third Avenue
New York, New York

June Halper, MSN, RN.CS, ANP
Executive Director, Gimbel MS Center
Consortium of Multiple Sclerosis Centers
Teaneck, New Jersey

T. Jock Murray, OC, MD, FRCPC, MACP
Director, Dalhousie MS Research Unit
Professor of Medical Humanities, Dalhousie University
Halifax, Nova Scotia

Aaron E. Miller, MD
Director, Division of Neurology
Maimonides Medical Center
4802 10th Avenue
Brooklyn, New York

Deborah P. Hertz, MPH
National Director of Medical Programs
National Multiple Sclerosis Society
New York, New York

CHAPTER 1

Multiple Sclerosis: The Disease and Its Diagnosis

Timothy L. Vollmer, MD

In 1868 Charcot provided a detailed description of the clinical and pathologic characteristics of multiple sclerosis (MS) (1). He described the
plaques of demyelination that characterize the disease and suggested that
a loss of myelin may play an important part in the pathophysiology of the
disorder. In 1933 Rivers and Schwentker described one of the first experimental models, experimental autoimmune encephalomyelitis (EAE), for
acute inflammatory demyelination (2). Experimental autoimmune
encephalomyelitis has been used extensively as a model of MS for immunologic, immunotherapeutic, and immunogenetic research. As a result, a
great deal has been learned about possible mechanisms underlying the
pathogenesis of MS. Although many questions remain, this work has resulted in three new immunologic therapies for MS being approved by the
Food and Drug Administration (FDA) for use in the United States since
1993, making MS one of the more treatable neurologic diseases (3,4,5)
(see Chapter 2).

EPIDEMIOLOGY

Multiple sclerosis is one of the leading causes of neurologic disability in
young adults. Currently, there are more than 400,000 patients with the
diagnosis of MS in North America. The disease generally has its onset in
the third or fourth decade, with more than 50 percent of patients beginning between the ages of 20 and 40. The risk of a first episode of MS peaks

at age 30 years. The initial presentation of MS in people younger than 10 years and older than 50 years accounts for less than 5 percent of cases. Age at onset does not show a strong correlation with geography or prevalence of the disease. Most studies show MS to be more common in women, with a female-male ratio between 1.4 and 2. Onset occurs at a slightly younger age in women (6,7).

Geographic factors are highly correlated with the risk of developing MS. In general, incidence and prevalence rates increase with increasing distance from the equator, both north and south. This pattern has been reported from all continents that have been studied, with the best studies carried out in North America, Europe, and Australia. For example, the crude prevalence of MS in Boston (latitude 41° N) is 120:100,000, compared with a crude prevalence of 50:100,000 in New Orleans (30° N). Superimposed on this global geographic pattern are occasional local "epidemics" of MS. Migration studies are also consistent with the hypothesis that risk of developing the disease is at least in part acquired on the basis of environmental conditions. Also, studies have suggested that the environmental factors that affect risk of developing MS act before age 15 years (8).

GENETICS

Multiple sclerosis prevalence rates are quite variable between different ethnic and racial groups, being highest in northern European Caucasians, with lower rates in African Americans and Asians. That at least some of the risk of developing MS is determined by genetic factors is supported by the increased concordance in identical twins (approximately 30 percent) as compared with fraternal twins (3 percent to 5 percent). In general, MS occurs in relatives of patients 10 to 50 times more often than in the general population. The absolute risk of first-degree relatives of MS patients is on average 2 percent to 5 percent, depending on the exact degree of relatedness (Table 1-1), as compared with an average risk in the general population of 0.1 percent (7,9). The basis of the association of risk with genetic factors is not yet well defined. However, it does appear that multiple genes are involved in determining risk.

VIROLOGY

Peripheral blood antibody titers to many viruses [e.g., measles, mumps, varicella zoster, vaccinia, rubella, human herpesvirus 6 (HHV-6), and Epstein-Barr virus] are elevated in people with MS. In some cases, virus-specific antibody is also detected in the cerebrospinal fluid (CSF) (10–12).

Table 1-1. Familial Risks for MS (Genetic Factors) (Ref. 67, 68)

⊃ Familial MS
  Up to 20 percent of MS subjects have at least one relative with MS
⊃ Empiric recurrence risks (age-adjusted)
  MS parent-risk for child: 4%
  MS subject-risk for sibling: 4%–5%
  MS twin with MS risk for co-twin (fraternal): 3%–5%
  MS twin with MS-risk for co-twin (identical): 26%–36%

Over the past several years, some investigators have found evidence of certain viral infections in the central nervous system (CNS) of MS patients and near MS plaques (e.g., HHV-6) (13). The relevance of these findings to the pathophysiology of the disease remains to be determined.

PATHOLOGY

Pathologically, MS is characterized by areas of focal demyelination (plaques) disseminated throughout the CNS in both space and time. As shown in Figures 1-1 and 1-2, the demyelinated plaques appear as lucent areas scattered in the central white matter, most commonly in the periventricular areas. Although the plaques may appear anywhere in the CNS,

Figure 1-1. Demyelination of white matter of cerebral hemispheres in MS. Note the extensive periventricular demyelination.

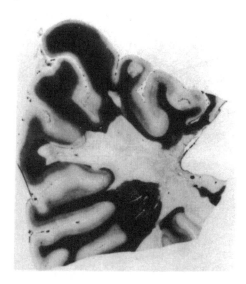

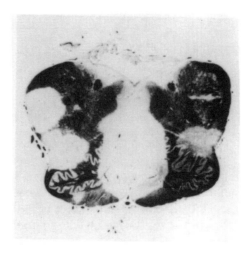

Figure 1-2. Multiple plaques in cerebellum and pons in MS.

and, in fact, often show a remarkable degree of dissemination, there is a predilection for the optic nerves and chiasm, spinal cord, brainstem, and cerebellar white matter. Plaques are occasionally also seen in gray matter.

Pathologic descriptions of demyelination may overstress the myelin-axonal dissociation: loss of myelin with preservation of axons. In fact, although loss of myelin is the most obvious finding in the MS plaque, it was pointed out by Adams and Kubik (14) in 1952 that some axons show gross degeneration. This observation has recently been extended by neuroimaging and pathologic studies showing that a subset of MS patients exhibit evidence of axonal destruction and that this subset has proportionately more disability (15,16).

Pathologic descriptions of MS have highlighted perivascular mononuclear cell infiltrates, frequently seen around postcapillary venules extending through the areas of demyelination. Eventually, the lymphocytic infiltrate fades, as do the macrophage and microglia infiltrates. These inflammatory infiltrates present in a "bursting" pattern, increasing and decreasing over variable periods of time, averaging approximately 6 weeks by magnetic resonance imaging (MRI) (17). The inflammatory activity recurs in the CNS such that patients with active MS can have several areas of active inflammation (indicated by gadolinium-enhancing lesions) on each cranial MRI performed on a monthly basis (18). Individual plaque appears to cycle through these episodes of inflammation independent of other areas of inflammation and demyelination in the patient's brain. The myelin-forming cells in the CNS, oligodendrocytes, are absent or reduced within the center of most plaques. However, there is some evidence of remyelination in early plaques

(19,20). Astrocytic proliferation is substantial and is responsible for the glial scarring that contributes the "sclerosis" to multiple sclerosis.

IMMUNOGENESIS

The cause of MS remains elusive. However, the evidence that the immune system plays a central role in the pathogenesis of the disease is overwhelming. From an MRI perspective, MS is a multiphasic disease, with each MS plaque in the CNS in its own phase of development. The inflammatory events are cyclic, with a predilection for recurrences to develop in areas previously attacked, resulting in the pulsatile growth of individual plaques over many years. Many MRI studies have shown that these inflammatory attacks on the CNS occur 5 to 12 times per year or more (Figure 1-3) (21,22).

Figure 1-3. Natural history of MS: MRI and clinical pattern. The relationship between frequency of MRI-detected inflammatory events (gadolinium-enhanced MRI), the progressive increase in MS plaque volume (MRI-detected burden of disease), cerebral atrophy, and neurologic impairment. As can be seen, exacerbations of neurologic impairment in MS are associated with a CNS inflammatory event. Most CNS inflammatory events, however, are not associated with a clear change in neurologic status. These inflammatory events do contribute to the total volume of demyelination, which correlates generally with progression of disability *(Adapted from Jerry S. Wolinsky, M.D.).*

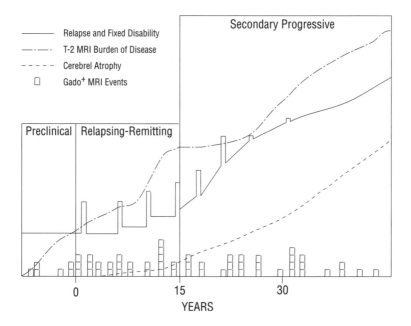

NATURAL HISTORY OF MS: MRI AND CLINICAL PATTERN

Although the majority of these events are clinically silent at the time of their development, they contribute to the burden of disease that does correlate with disability (23).

Attacks of MS can be provoked by febrile illness, most of which are viral upper respiratory tract infections (24). Also, the first 6 months after pregnancy (post partum) are associated with an increased risk of MS exacerbation (25). However, the factors that provoke an inflammatory attack on the CNS are not known in a majority of cases. Regardless of what initiates the inflammatory disease, there is transmigration of autoaggressive T lymphocytes into the brain. The biology of the migration of peripheral lymphocytes across endothelial cells of the blood–brain barrier has been dramatically elucidated by recent work (26). Thus a number of potential targets for therapeutic intervention have been identified in MS.

The actual molecular target of the immune attack (if any) in MS is not known. A similar disease (EAE) can be initiated in rodents and primates using purified myelin basic protein (MBP), proteolipid protein (PLP), and myelin oligodendrocyte glycoprotein (MOG) (27–33). Myelin basic protein–reactive T cells with a memory phenotype can be isolated from patients with MS (29,31). The mechanisms that lead directly to myelin destruction in an MS plaque are not known (34). However, tumor necrosis factor (TNF) produced by activated T lymphocytes and other cells (including astrocytes) has been shown to induce apoptosis in oligodendrocytes (35).

NEUROPHYSIOLOGY

A large body of evidence shows that focal demyelination causes slowed conduction, a failure to transmit high-frequency trains of impulses, or a total conduction block (36,37). Clearly, such changes will result in neurologic dysfunction, although its actual clinical expression is difficult to predict. Demyelinated fibers under experimental circumstances show ectopic impulse generation, increased sensitivity to mechanical distortion, and abnormal interactions between fibers ("cross-talk") (38–40). These conduction abnormalities may underlie the "positive" signs and symptoms in demyelinating disease such as Lhermitte's sign, various pain syndromes, and tonic flexor spasms.

Demyelinated fibers exhibit a heightened sensitivity to internal milieu: to temperature and to the makeup of the ionic environment (41–43). This is due to the fact that the safety factor in demyelinated fibers is reduced, often to a value of one or lower, compared with a value of approximately six in normal myelinated fibers. Axons with low safety factors are very sensitive to small changes in excitability. A frequent observation in MS patients is that clinical deficits worsen, or latent deficits become manifest, when body temperature is elevated (44–46). Alkalosis, which is known to increase axonal excitability, may be accompanied by conduction in axons previously exhibiting conduction block. This variability of conduction and increased sensitivity to exogenous conditions may provide a partial explanation for the symptoms that often appear and disappear within a rapid time course in MS.

CLINICAL SIGNS AND SYMPTOMS

Given the varied nature and distribution of pathologic lesions in MS, it is expected that the disease will present a variety of clinical deficits or combinations of deficits. McAlpine and colleagues (47) reported that the incidence of initial symptoms (occurring alone or in combination with other symptoms) is as follows: motor weakness in one or more limbs, 40 percent; optic neuritis, 22 percent; paresthesia and other sensory disturbances, 21 percent; diplopia, 12 percent; vertigo or vomiting, 5 percent; disturbances of bladder function, 5 percent.

Table 1-2 is derived from 55 sequential patients with MS from our own experience. It shows the frequency of various signs and symptoms at the time of diagnosis and within 5 years of onset of symptoms. Multiple sclerosis often presents with an asymmetric distribution of clinical deficits early in the course. In most patients, however, as MS worsens, lesions become distributed on both sides of the neuraxis and there is a tendency to bilateral disability. A unilateral deficit seen in later stages of the disease weighs against the diagnosis of MS.

Table 1-2. Signs and Symptoms in 55 Patients with Probable or Definite MS

Disturbance	At Diagnosis		Within 5 years	
	No.	%	No.	%
Spasticity/paresis	17	31	43	78
Sensory disorder	21	38	45	82
Visual loss	16	29	29	53
Diplopia	9	16	14	26
Brainstem signs	13	24	39	71
Ataxia	8	15	33	60
Sphincter dysfunction	5	9	23	42
Altered mental status	2	4	7	13

Fatigue

Fatigue is the most common symptom reported by MS patients, with up to 90 percent of patients reporting it at one time or another during the course of their disease (see Chapter 3). It does not necessarily correlate with the severity or activity of an individual's MS. It may be described as lassitude or lack of energy, somnolence, or lethargy. It also is expressed as easy fatigability during exercise such as prolonged ambulation, manifesting as an increasing sensation of heaviness and weakness in the legs. Fatigue is one of the most disabling symptoms of MS.

Depression

Depression is the second most common symptom of MS. Like fatigue, depression does not correlate with the severity of the neurologic disease in either severity or frequency. Also, it is more common in MS than in other chronic illnesses. As many as 70 percent of MS patients will report symptoms of depression at some time during the course of their disease. Like fatigue, depression contributes to the "invisible" disability of MS.

Visual Involvement

Abnormalities of vision are common in many patients with MS (see also Chapter 8). These abnormalities most commonly result from plaques forming in the optic nerve or chiasm, but may also result from damage to the optic tract or radiation. Even patients who do not have a clinically detectable visual deficit often have abnormalities of visual pathways that can be demonstrated electrophysiologically. Some patients may describe visual "blurring" or "haziness," which may resolve rapidly, stabilize, or progress to complete visual loss in the affected eye. Periorbital pain may occur before visual failure by hours or a few days. The visual fields often demonstrate a central or paracentral scotoma, which may be especially well delineated when a small (3 mm) red object is used for testing. Some degree of pupillary dilation, a sluggish response to light, and a Marcus Gunn pupil (demonstrated by the "swinging flashlight" test: pupillary dilation is seen when a light is moved from the unaffected to the affected side) are often seen. Ophthalmoscopic examination may reveal optic pallor, which can progress to the "chalk white" discs of pronounced optic atrophy.

Optic neuritis is often the presenting episode of MS, but not all patients with optic neuritis develop classic MS. Estimates of the probability of developing MS after a bout of optic neuritis vary from 15 percent to 85 percent. An abnormal cranial MRI with "silent" plaques in patients with idiopathic optic neuritis increases the subsequent risk of MS to as high as 90 percent (23).

Motor Symptoms

Motor involvement may occur quite early in the course of MS, especially in patients who present with multiple symptoms (see Chapter 4). The patient may initially complain of ill-defined "weakness" or "heaviness" in an affected limb, or may describe a tendency to trip or fall, or to drag the affected leg. Involvement of the pyramidal tracts, either in the spinal cord or higher in the CNS, produces weakness typical of an upper motor neuron lesion. Consequently, the clinical picture often includes spasticity, hyperreflexia, clonus, and extensor plantar responses. Muscle contractures may occur in patients with advanced disease. Fasciculations are not seen. Muscle wasting, when observed, is due to disuse and not to lower motor neuron pathology. Involvement of the corticobulbar tracts bilaterally occurs in some patients and leads to a pseudobulbar state characterized by dysarthria, dysphagia, hyperactive jaw jerk, bifacial plegia, and apparent emotional lability (a dissociation between subjective affective state and pathologic crying or laughing is a hallmark of pseudobulbar palsy).

Sensory Symptoms

Many patients complain of vague and poorly characterized sensory symptoms. These can be transient, appearing and remitting within a rapid time course, sometimes less than 24 hours. Some patients complain of a sensation of "squeezing," "burning," or "pressure" in a bandlike distribution around the thorax, indicating a plaque in the spinal cord. In other cases, the patient may complain of numbness or paresthesias over the limbs, sometimes mimicking disease of the peripheral nervous system. The radiation of tingling or electric-like paresthesias into the limbs or trunk on flexion of the neck is reported by many patients and is referred to as Lhermitte's sign, which reflects involvement of the cervical spinal cord.

Sensory signs on neurologic examination may initially be slight in degree and difficult to demonstrate. Superficial sensation to pin prick, thermal sense, or light touch, may be impaired in an area roughly contiguous to the region of subjective sensory abnormality. Vibratory sensibility and joint position sense are often dissociated, with propioception more often being abnormal. In some cases with plaques in the spinal cord, a distinct sensory level may be found. "Sensory ataxia" may become manifest either in gait or in clumsiness of fine movements of the upper extremity, and may lead to a loss of dexterity in the face of relatively preserved strength.

Brainstem Symptoms

The more common clinical abnormalities include ophthalmoplegia, especially internuclear ophthalmoplegia (weakness of adduction with nystagmus of the abducting eye on lateral gaze, presumably due to involvement of the medial longitudinal fasciculus) and nystagmus. Nystagmus occurs in more than one half of MS patients. Horizontal nystagmus on lateral gaze is most common, but a rotatory component may be present even early in the course of the disease. Vertical nystagmus is less common but is associated with demyelinating lesions of the brainstem.

Vertigo occurs as an initial symptom in approximately 5 percent of patients. During the course of the disease, vertigo may occur in as many as 40 percent to 50 percent of patients (see Chapter 4); in many patients vomiting accompanies the vertigo.

Facial numbness, weakness, or pain are less common, but they do occur. Paroxysmal unilateral facial pain occurs in approximately 2 percent of patients. "Trigger zones" are less commonly present than in the idiopathic form of trigeminal neuralgia. The diagnosis of MS should be considered in all patients under age 50 years presenting with a picture of trigeminal neuralgia.

Facial weakness, often of a peripheral type, may occur in as many as 5 percent of patients with MS. The lack of pain and preservation of taste distinguish this from Bell's palsy. Hemifacial spasm or facial myokymia may also occur, although neither of these is pathognomonic for MS. Deafness is uncommon, probably as a result of the bilateral routing of sensory signals for this sense.

Cerebellar Involvement

The relatively common involvement of cerebellar systems in MS was emphasized by Charcot. Intention tremor is often seen and may be disabling (see Chapter 4). Truncal ataxia and ataxia of gait are often present. Dysarthria is seen in many patients due, at least in part, to ataxia of the muscles controlling articulation, although pseudobulbar weakness may also contribute. "Scanning" speech, characterized by dyssynergic articulation, is often present and is highly characteristic of cerebellar involvement in the disease.

Genitourinary and Bowel Symptoms

Bladder symptoms are almost universal in the later stages of MS (see Chapter 6). The initial presentation includes bladder problems in at least 5 percent; in some cases, bladder dysfunction may constitute the only initial symptom. Urinary urgency, often coupled with frequency, is the most common early genitourinary problem. Incontinence may occur. Uninhibited neurogenic bladder, resulting from a spinal cord lesion above S1, begins with overflow incontinence that evolves into bladder automaticity. Urinary hesitancy or retention is also reported by some patients but is less common. In many patients, the bladder is never completely emptied and urinary tract infections are not uncommon. Approximately 50 percent of male patients experience sexual problems (usually impotence) at some time during the course of their disease.

Bowel dysfunction is seen in approximately 60 percent of MS patients (see Chapter 7). Both constipation and involuntary bowel action may occur, with constipation being by far the more frequent. In addition to neurogenic etiology, constipation may have many causes, including medications used to treat other MS-related problems, inadequate fluid intake, insufficient dietary bulk, decreased mobility, and spasticity.

Higher Cortical Function

Changes in higher cortical function are common, occurring in approximately 40 percent of MS patients. The most common complaints relate to short-term memory dysfunction, difficulty in managing complex tasks, and confusion. Frank dementia is rare but may occur in patients with aggressive forms of MS.

Tonic Spasms

Tonic flexion spasms, which consist of brief increases in flexor tone in one or more limbs, often associated with a great deal of pain, occur in some patients with MS (see Chapter 4). These spasms are presumably due to abnormalities in the spinal cord (48), although the precise cause is not clear. Attacks of paroxysmal dysarthria sometimes associated with ataxia and lasting for minutes have also been described (49).

Suicide

Suicide can be considered a "symptom" of MS because the risk of suicide in MS patients is 7.5 times increased as compared with the general population. The clinician must actively seek evidence of suicidal thoughts and behavior if he is to have a chance of intervening before a tragedy occurs.

COURSE AND PROGNOSIS

Despite its unpredictability, the course of MS may be classified as four types. These types have been defined by an international survey of MS experts:

- ⊃ *Relapsing-Remitting*—This is the classic form of the disease, presenting in 85 percent of MS patients at onset. In relapsing-remitting MS, relapses are clearly distinguished from periods of remission, during which the symptoms resolve or partially resolve. It is not unusual, however, for each relapse to leave an increasing degree of fixed clinical deficit. The periods between disease relapses are characterized by a lack of disease progression.

- ⊃ *Secondary Progressive*—From 50 percent to 70 percent of the patients who initially present with relapsing-remitting MS eventually develop secondary progressive MS. In this form patients may continue to have relapses, but in addition they note a slow steady loss of neurologic function only recognized in retrospect (50).

- ⊃ *Progressive-Relapsing*—Approximately 5 percent of patients have progressive-relapsing MS. This pattern of MS shows progression from onset, with clear, acute relapses that may or may not resolve with full recovery.

- ⊃ *Primary Progressive*—The remaining 10 percent of MS patients have primary progressive MS. The disease shows a nearly continuous worsening from its onset, without distinct relapses and remissions or occasional plateaus and temporary minor improvements. It is more commonly seen in people who develop the disease after the age of 40 years.

Whether these clinical classifications are significant in terms of selection of immunologic therapies remains to be determined. However, because these clinical definitions are used to select patients for clinical trials, the FDA often approves the use of new immunologic therapies only in the clinical subtypes of MS studied. In the author's opinion, there is no compelling evidence that these clinical definitions identify variations in pathophysiology or response to immunologic therapies. Therefore, such classifications should not be overemphasized in the clinical management of MS patients (51).

The clinical characteristics of early disease that may have prognostic significance are listed in Table 1-3. However, the power of these clinical observations in early disease to predict future outcome in MS is weak. Magnetic resonance imaging has become a useful prognostic tool

Table 1-3. Clinical Factors with Prognostic Value in MS

Favorable	Unfavorable
Younger age at onset	Older age at onset
Female	Male
Normal MRI at presentation	High lesion load on MRI at presentation
Complete recovery from first relapse	Lack of recovery from first relapse
Low relapse rate	High relapse rate
	Early cerebellar involvement
Long interval to second relapse	Short interval to second relapse
Low disability at 2 and 4 years	Early development of mild disability
	Insidious motor onset

(17,18,23). Magnetic resonance imaging and/or MR spectroscopy may be able to determine the amount of axonal destruction occurring in MS as well, which should further refine our prognostic ability (16). However, benign MS (defined as an Expanded Disability Status Score—EDSS—of less than 3.5 after at least 15 years of disease) occurs in less than 20 percent of MS patients (7). Therefore, at the time of diagnosis, the physician may anticipate that 8 of 10 newly diagnosed MS patients face at least moderate disability that will negatively impact their family, career, and general health (7). Without treatment, at least 50 percent of MS patients will be using a cane or other device to assist their ambulation within 15 years of onset of the disease and one third will ultimately require the use of a wheelchair. From the standpoint of family and career, however, the less visible symptoms of fatigue, depression, pain, and cognitive dysfunction are also important (50,52). Therefore, *the* challenge to the clinician is not to identify those patients with a poor prognosis, but rather to identify the few patients whose MS is likely to be so benign that the currently available therapies have little to offer. The brain MRI appears to be particularly powerful when used to identify those individuals with a high likelihood of benign MS (23).

DIAGNOSIS

Schumacher and colleagues (53) listed six diagnostic criteria for MS:

1. Evidence, on neurologic examination or by history, of involvement of two or more sites in the CNS ("lesions separated in space")
2. Involvement of the CNS in one of the following temporal patterns: two or more distinct periods of worsening separated by a time period of 1 month or more, each lasting at least 24 hours; or a slow or

stepwise progression over a course of at least 6 months ("lesions separated in time")
3. Objective abnormalities on neurologic examination referable to dysfunction of the CNS
4. Evidence that CNS disease reflects primarily disease of the white matter
5. Onset between the age of 10 years and 50 years
6. A decision that the patient's signs and symptoms cannot better be explained by another diagnosis after a thorough neurologic evaluation

These criteria can assist in diagnosing the majority of MS patients, but some patients, particularly at onset of disease, may not manifest all these characteristics. Also, MS can present before the age of 10 years and after the age of 50 years. In the pre-MRI era, patients were followed up, sometimes for years, to allow the disease to clearly manifest all of the aforementioned characteristics before a final diagnosis was made, during which time the patient often accumulated significant disability. This approach is no longer viable with advent of the newer immunologic therapies, which should be started as early as possible in the disease course of most patients. Thus, the brain and spine MRI have become the most important diagnostic tests to ascertain or confirm "lesions consistent with demyelination disseminated in both space and time." Cerebrospinal fluid examination also plays an important role in the diagnosis of MS.

DIFFERENTIAL DIAGNOSIS

The initial presentation of MS is protean in its variety. Neurologic diseases that are commonly confused with MS include spinal cord compression from tumor or spondylosis, platybasia, basilar impression, Arnold-Chiari malformation, intracranial tumor, CNS lymphoma, vasculitis of the CNS, acute disseminated encephalomyelitis, transverse myelitis, neurosyphilis, neuro-Lyme disease, vitamin B12 deficiency, heredodegenerative disease such as Friedreich's ataxia and the spinocerebellar degenerations, Leber's optic atrophy, and motor neuron disease.

LABORATORY FINDINGS

In view of the difficulties that may be encountered in making the clinical diagnosis of MS, numerous laboratories have devoted considerable effort to the development of tests to aid in diagnosis. These tests are often of con-

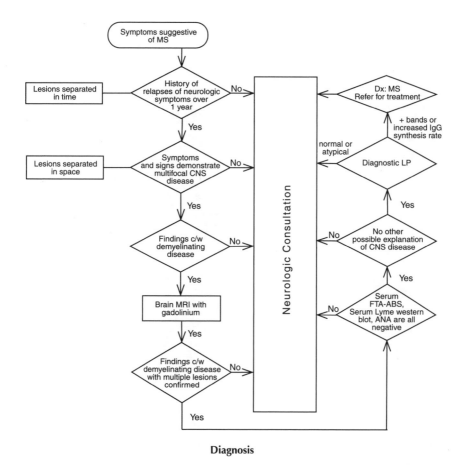

Diagnosis

siderable use. However, no single test has yet been devised by which the diagnosis can be made with confidence in 100 percent of patients. Especially in the case of a disease with as variable a course as MS, laboratory findings must be interpreted in the light of the clinical picture.

Magnetic Resonance Imaging

Magnetic resonance imaging (MRI) has a high degree of specificity and sensitivity in detecting demyelination in the cerebral hemispheres (Figure 1-4) (54). Magnetic resonance imaging can quantitate the volume of disease involving the CNS and lesions, and during acute attacks MRI can be correlated with clinical symptoms (55–59). Longitudinal studies reveal that the bulk of lesions are clinically silent and that many lesions may come and go on serial MRIs (60–62), thus demonstrating that the clinical examina-

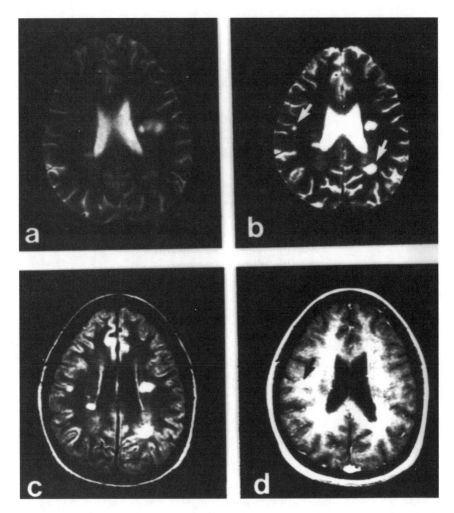

Figure 1-4. Magnetic resonance imaging from a 26-year-old woman with a 2-year history of laboratory-supported definite MS. Her only new symptom is decreased vision in both eyes, which began 4 months before this study and may be explained by the left occipital lesion. Note the gadolinium-enhancing lesion in the left parietal area, which represents a currently active but asymptomatic lesion.

tion is relatively insensitive in detecting pathologic progression in early disease.

The introduction of contrast-enhancing agents with MRI allowed the identification of areas of blood–brain barrier breakdown (55,63). These areas correlate with active inflammatory demyelination (17,18). The volume of disease as measured by quantitative MRI analysis correlates with disease severity but only moderately. It is not surprising that the correlation of the MRI and clinical disability is not strong because there are at least three variables to consider when extrapolating from MRI images to the patient in terms of MS.

⊃ The first variable is the total volume of MS plaque (23).

⊃ The second variable is the location of the disease. Clearly, brainstem, optic nerve, and spinal cord disease has more impact on the neurologic examination than cerebral disease.

⊃ Third, we need to know the impact of the inflammatory process on the integrity of the axon. Recent studies suggest that there may be a subset of MS patients who suffer substantial axonal loss and secondary neuronal loss in addition to demyelination. These patients suffer significant cerebral atrophy, have more significant abnormalities on magnetic resonance spectroscopic analysis of the "normal appearing white matter," and have more pronounced plague signals on a T-1 weighted MRI of the cerebral hemispheres (15). The immunologic basis for this finding remains to be elucidated. Magnetic resonance imaging thus allows the assessment of disease severity, disease activity, and disease progression.

Cerebrospinal Fluid

Abnormal intrathecal antibody production, detected as oligoclonal immunoglobulin, was one of the earliest immune abnormalities identified in MS. More than 90 percent of patients with clinically definite MS will have oligoclonal immunoglobulin and/or elevated immunoglobulin levels in the CSF (64,65). The CSF glucose level is normal. The CSF protein level is usually normal but may be mildly elevated; values above 100 mg are rarely seen and should lead to a reevaluation of the diagnosis. Mild increases in the CSF cell count are common. These are usually on the order of 5 to 10 mononuclear cells/mm^3, although up to 100 mononuclear cells/mm^3 may be seen.

The utility of CSF examination in MS is to confirm by the presence of oligoclonal immunoglobulin that the suspected CNS disease is a chronic inflammatory one. The sensitivity of the test from this point of view is approximately 50 percent in new onset MS, but it increases to approximately 90 percent in MS of at least 2 years duration. It also is useful in identifying many of the diseases that mimic MS (i.e., CSF VDRL, CSF Lyme western blot assay, cytology).

Evoked Potentials

Evoked potentials (EPs) are useful in confirming "lesions of the white matter separated in space." The stimulus used for visual evoked potentials

(VEPs) in most laboratories consists of a reversing "checkerboard" pattern, with the cortical signals recorded by surface electrode over the occiput. Prolonged latencies, in some cases with a reduction in amplitude, are seen in the majority of patients with demyelination of the visual pathway. It should be emphasized that delayed visual evoked responses, although common in MS, also occur in other disorders. These include spinocerebellar degenerations, congenital optic atrophies, and compressive lesions involving the visual pathways. Nevertheless, assessment of visual evoked responses is extremely useful because it allows the noninvasive evaluation of conduction latency along the visual pathway.

Multiphasic peaks (labeled I to VII by most workers) in response to an auditory stimulus such as a monaural click are detected in response to a brainstem auditory evoked potential (BAEP) examination. These peaks appear to reflect activity in the eighth cranial nerve, cochlear nucleus, superior olivary complex, tracts or nuclei of lateral lemniscus, inferior colliculus, and possibly the medial geniculate body, auditory radiations, and temporal lobe. Somatosensory evoked responses are elicited by electrical stimulus applied to the extremities and subsequent neural signals recorded from the scalp.

Although clinically silent abnormalities may be detected with all the modalities of evoked response (visual, somatosensory, brainstem, auditory), it is interesting that this more commonly occurs in the visual pathway. Thus, despite the fact that the spinal pathway is longer (and therefore might be expected to be involved more frequently if lesions were randomly distributed throughout the neuraxis), clinically silent lesions are more commonly demonstrated by VEPs (66). Evoked potentials as a diagnostic aid in MS have largely been replaced by cranial MRI.

Serologies and Blood Studies

Blood studies in MS patients are generally normal. Therefore, any significant abnormalities on general chemistry, hematologic, and urine screens may suggest an alternative diagnosis and should be pursued. Serum assays for syphilis, Lyme disease, and collagen vascular diseases should be considered in the evaluation of possible MS.

SUMMARY

Multiple sclerosis is one of the most common major neurologic diseases to afflict young adults in North America and many other parts of the world. Using modern diagnostic aids in conjunction with a thorough neurologic evaluation, the diagnosis can be made early in almost all patients. Early diagnosis is a key to timely intervention with the currently available immunologic therapies. It also avoids the anxious and depressing uncertainty or misdiagnosis that so many MS patients have suffered as a result of delays in the diagnosis of their disease.

REFERENCES

1. Charcot JM. Histologie de la sclerose en plaques. *Gaz Hop (Paris)* 1868:454.
2. Rivers T, Schwentker F. Encephalomyelitis accompanied by myelin destruction experimentally produced in monkeys. *J Exp Med* 1935; 61:689.
3. Paty DW, Li DKB. Interferon beta-1b is effective in relapsing-remitting multiple sclerosis. *Neurology* 1993; 43:662–667.
4. Jacobs LD, et al. Intramuscular interferon beta-1a for disease progression in relapsing multiple sclerosis. *Ann Neurol* 1996; 39(3):285–294.
5. Johnson KP, et al. Copolymer 1 reduces relapse rate and improves disability in relapsing-remitting multiple sclerosis: Results of phase III multicenter, double-blind placebo-controlled trial. *Neurology* 1995; 45(7):1268–1276.
6. Kurland LT. The epidemiological characteristics of multiple sclerosis. *Handbook of neurology.* Amsterdam: North Holland, 1970.
7. Weinschenker BG. Epidemiology of multiple sclerosis. *Neurol Clin* 1996; 14(2):291–308.
8. Dean G, Kurtzke J. A critical age for the acquisition of multiple sclerosis. *Trans Am Neurol Assoc* 1970; 95:232.
9. Oksenberg JR, Seboun E, Hauser SL. Genetics of demyelinating diseases. *Brain Pathol* 1996; 6(3):289–302.
10. Brody JA, Sever JL, Edgar A, et al. Measles antibody titers of multiple sclerosis patients and their siblings. *Neurology (Minneap)* 1970; 22:492.
11. Symington GR, MacKay IR, Whittingham S, et al. A "profile" of immune responsiveness in multiple sclerosis. *Clin Exp Immunol* 1978; 31:141.
12. Johnson KP, Likosky WP, Nelson BJ, et al. Comprehensive viral immunology of multiple sclerosis. *Arch Neurol* 1980; 37:537.
13. Liedtke W, Malessa R, Faustmann PM, et al. Human herpesvirus 6 polymerase chain reaction findings in human immunodeficiency virus associated neurological disease and multiple sclerosis. *J Neurovirol* 1995; 1:253–238.
14. Adams RD, Kubik C. Morbid anatomy of the demyelinative diseases. *Am J Med* 1952; 12:510.
15. Van Walderveen M, et al. Histopathologic correlate of hypointense lesions on T1-weighted SE MR images in multiple sclerosis. *Neurology* 1997; 48:A360–361.
16. Trapp BD, Peterson J, Ransohoff RM, et al. Axonal transection in the lesions of multiple sclerosis. *N Engl J Med* 1998; 338:278–285.
17. Stone LA, et al. Blood–brain barrier disruption on contrast-enhanced MRI in patients with mild relapsing-remitting multiple sclerosis: Relationship to course, gender and age. *Neurology* 1995; 45(6):1122–1126.
18. Stone LA, et al. Changes in the amount of diseased white matter over time in patients with relapsing-remitting multiple sclerosis. *Neurology* 1995a; 45(10):1808–1814.

19. Aravella LS, Herndon RM. Mature oligodendrocytes: Division following experimental demyelination in adult animals. *Arch Neurol* 1984; 41:1162.
20. Ludwin SK. Remyelination in the central nervous system and the peripheral nervous system. *Advances in Neurology: Functional recovery in neurological disease.* New York: Raven Press, 1988:47.
21. Smith ME, et al. Clinical worsening in multiple sclerosis is associated with increased frequency and area of gadopentetate dimeglumine–enhancing magnetic resonance imaging lesions. *Ann Neurol* 1993; 33(5):480–489.
22. Thompson AJ, Kermode AG, Wicks D. Major differences in the dynamics of primary and secondary progressive multiple sclerosis. *Ann Neurol* 1991; 29:53–62.
23. Filippi M, et al. Quantitative brain MRI lesion load predicts the course of clinically isolated syndromes suggestive of multiple sclerosis. *Neurology* 1994; 44:635–641.
24. Sibley WA, Bamford CR, Clark K. Clinical viral infections and multiple sclerosis. *Lancet* 1985; 1:1313–1315.
25. Abramsky O. Pregnancy and multiple sclerosis. *Ann Neurol* 1994; 36:S38–S41.
26. Cannella B, Raine CS. The adhesion molecule and cytokine profile of multiple sclerosis lesions. *Ann Neurol* 1995; 37(4):424–435.
27. Kies MW. Species-specificity and localization of encephalitogenic sites in myelin basic protein. *Spr Sem Immunopathol* 1985; 8:295.
28. Zamvil SS, et al. T-cell epitope of the autoantigen myelin basic protein that induces encephalomyelitis. *Nature* 1986; 324:258.
29. Kono DH, et al. Two minor determinants of myelin basic protein induce experimental allergic encephalomyelitis in SJL/J mice. *J Exp Med* 1988; 168:213.
30. Rechert JR, et al. Fine specifications of myelin basic protein-specific human T-cell clones. *Ann NY Acad Sci* 1988; 540:345.
31. Satoh J, Koike F, Tabira T. Experimental allergic encephalomyelitis mediated by murine encephalitogenic T-cell lines specific for myelin proteolipid apoprotein. *Ann NY Acad Sci* 1988; 540:343.
32. Barevanis CN, Relos GJ, Sewis C, et al. Peptides of myelin basic protein stimulate thymocytes from patients with multiple sclerosis. *J Immunol* 1989; 22(1):23.
33. Kusunoki S, Yu RK, Kim JH. Introduction of experimental allergic encephalomyelitis in guinea pigs using myelin basic protein and myelin glycolipids. *J Neuroimmunol* 1988; 18(4):303.
34. Raine C. The immunology of the multiple sclerosis lesion. *Ann Neurol* 1994; 36:S61–S72.
35. Paul NL, Ruddle NH. Lymphotoxin. *Ann Rev Immunol* 1988; 6:407.
36. McDonald WI. Pathophysiology of multiple sclerosis. *Brain* 1974; 87:179.
37. Waxman SG. Clinicopathological correlations in multiple sclerosis and related diseases. *Demyelinating diseases: Clinical and basic electrophysiology.* New York: Raven Press, 1981:169–182.
38. Rasminsky M. *Pathophysiology of conduction in demyelinated axons.* New York: Raven Press, 1978:361–376.
39. Burchiel K. Abnormal impulse generation in focally demyelinated trigeminal roots. *J Neurosurg* 1980; 53:674–683.
40. Smith KJ, McDonald WI. Spontaneous and mechanically evoked activity due to central demyelinating lesions. *Nature* 1980; 286:154–155.

41. Becker FO, Michael JA, Davis FA. Acute effects of oral phosphate on visual function in multiple sclerosis. *Neurology* (Minneap) 1974; 24:601.
42. Davis FA, Becker FO, Michael JA, et al. Effects of intravenous sodium bicarbonate, disodium edetate (Na2EDTA) and hyperventilation on visual and oculomotor signs in multiple sclerosis. *J Neurol Neurosurg Psychiatry* 1970; 33:723.
43. Schauf CL, Davis FA. Impulse conduction in multiple sclerosis: A theoretical basis for modification by temperature and pharmacological agents. *J Neurol Neurosurg Psychiatry 1974; 37:152.*
44. Davis FA, Michael JA, Neer D. Serial hyperthermia testing in multiple sclerosis. *Acta Neurol Scand* 1973; 49:63.
45. Waxman SG. Clinical course and electrophysiology of multiple sclerosis. *Functional recovery in neurological disease.* New York: Raven Press, 1988:157–184.
46. Rasminsky, M. The effects of temperature on conduction in demyelinated single nerve fibers. *Arch Neurol* 1973; 28:287.
47. McAlpine D, Lumsden CE, Acheson ED. *Multiple sclerosis: A reappraisal.* London: Churchill Livingstone, 1972.
48. Matthews W. Tonic seizures in disseminated sclerosis. *Brain* 1958; 81:193.
49. Espir M, Watkins T, Smith H. Paroxysmal dysarthria and other transient neurological disturbances in disseminated sclerosis. *J Neurol Neurosurg Psychiatry 1966; 29:323.*
50. Confavreux C, Aimand G, Devic M. The course and prognosis of multiple sclerosis assessed by the computerized data processing of 349 patients. *Brain* 1980; 103:281.
51. Goodkin DE, Rudick RA, Hertsgaard D. Exacerbation rates and adherence to disease type in prospectively followed multiple sclerosis population: Implications for clinical trials. *Neurology* 1989; 39:357.
52. Poser S. *Multiple sclerosis: An analysis of 812 cases by means of electronic data processing.* Berlin: Springer-Verlag, 1978.
53. Schumacher G, Beebe G, Kibler R, et al. Problems of experimental trials of therapy in multiple sclerosis: Report by the panel on the evaluation of experimental trials on therapy in multiple sclerosis. *Ann NY Acad Sci* 1965; 1:552.
54. Farlow MR, et al. Multiple sclerosis: Magnetic resonance imaging, evoked responses, and spinal fluid electrophoresis. *Neurology* 1986; 36:828.
55. Miller DH, Rudge P, Johnson G, et al. Serial gadolinium enhanced magnetic resonance imaging in multiple sclerosis. *Brain* 1988; 111:927.
56. Paty DW, et al. MRI in the diagnosis of multiple sclerosis: A prospective study with comparison of clinical evaluation, evoked potentials, oligoclonal banding, and CT. *Neurology* 1988; 38:180.
57. Edwards MK, Farlow MR, Stevens JC. Multiple sclerosis: MRI and clinical correlation. *Am J Radiol* 1986; 147:571.
58. Koopmans RA, et al. Benign versus chronic progressive multiple sclerosis: Magnetic resonance imaging features. *Ann Neurol* 1989; 25(1):74.
59. Ormerod IEC, Miller DH, McDonald WI, et al. The role of NMR imaging in the assessment of multiple sclerosis and isolated neurological lesions. *Brain* 1987; 110:1579.
60. Ormerod IEC, McDonald WI, du Boulay GH, et al. Disseminated lesions at presentation in patients with optic neuritis. *J Neurol Neurosurg Psychiatry* 1986; 49:124.

61. Willoughby EW, et al. Serial magnetic resonance scanning in multiple sclerosis: A second prospective study in relapsing patients. *Ann Neurol* 1989; 25(1):43.
62. Issac C, et al. Multiple sclerosis: A serial study using MRI in relapsing patients. *Neurology* 1988; 38:1511.
63. Grossman RI, et al. Multiple sclerosis: Serial study of gadolinium-enhanced MR imaging. *Radiology* 1988; 169:117.
64. Hosein ZZ, Johnson KP. Isoelectric focusing of cerebrospinal fluid proteins in the diagnosis of multiple sclerosis. *Neurology* 1981; 31:70.
65. Johnson KP. Cerebrospinal fluid and blood assays of diagnostic usefulness in multiple sclerosis. *Neurology* (Minneap) 1980a; 30:106.
66. Hume AL, Waxman SG. Evoked potentials in suspected multiple sclerosis: Diagnostic value and prediction of clinical course. *J Neurol Sci* 1988; 83:191.
67. Sadovnick AD, Baird PA, Ward RH. Multiple sclerosis: Updated risks for relatives. *Am J Med Genet* 1988; 29:533–541.
68. Sadovnick AD, Armstrong H, Rice GP, et al. A population-based study of multiple sclerosis in twins: Update. *Ann Neurol* 1993; 33:281–285.

CHAPTER 2

Treatments to Reduce Disease Progression and Disability

Stanley van den Noort, MD

When a diagnosis of multiple sclerosis (MS) has been made, we need to move on to management strategies. These strategies include the management of symptoms (discussed in Chapters 3 to 10), the management of acute attacks, and the use of recently developed therapies to minimize disease progression. The relationship between the patient and the treating physician will be an ongoing one, as with any chronic disease, and this relationship must be based on mutual trust. When a firm diagnosis or even a working diagnosis of MS is made, it is therefore important to:

➲ Tell the patient the truth.

➲ Educate the patient about the complex and unpredictable nature of this disease, which does not usually shorten life span but may produce some degree of disability over the years.

➲ Refer the patient to information and support sources such as the National Multiple Sclerosis Society.

➲ Tell the patient that you will remain available for continuing care and support.

➲ Inform the patient of current treatments to treat attacks and reduce relapses.

People with MS have a complex unpredictable disease that proceeds over decades to produce symptoms that impact wellness, independence, careers, and families. They need a lot of time-intensive help from medical professionals, which should be educational and supportive. Many symptomatic and rehabilitative measures, which are discussed in other chapters, are critically important to permit life to continue in an acceptable way. This chapter deals with the treatment of acute relapses and treatments to slow disease progression and the accumulation of disability.

Multiple sclerosis is a confusing disease. An onset or worsening of symptoms is not always an attack, and worsening of disability is not always disease progression. An "attack" may actually be a pseudoexacerbation and may reflect an infection, exhaustion, a failure in coping mechanisms, or depression. "Progression" may be due not to increased disease activity but rather to decreased exercise, failure of environmental supports, depression, or similar problems. Paroxysmal symptoms that last seconds or minutes and are marked by pain, weakness, ataxia, vertigo, or dysarthria are not uncommon and do not necessarily represent disease progression.

Multiple sclerosis is characterized as relapsing-remitting, secondary progressive, primary progressive, or progressive-relapsing. In its most common form—relapsing-remitting disease—(which affects approximately 85 percent at onset), the illness begins with attacks of highly variable severity that generally occur from one to three times a year; attacks last from one to 90 days; spontaneous recovery from attacks may be dramatic and complete or slow and incomplete. Over a decade, attack frequency generally declines. A transition to secondary progressive disease is common but may not appear for several decades. Primary progressive MS represents approximately 10 percent of cases, some of which are actually secondary progressive patients who deny, suppress, or forget earlier symptoms. Perhaps 5 percent are progressive-relapsing, although this form of MS is controversial.

There are now accepted treatments for acute attacks and for reducing the frequency and severity of attacks. There is growing consensus that agents that reduce attack frequency also slow the progression of disability and that secondary progressive MS also responds to these agents. Magnetic resonance imaging (MRI) studies show that acute attacks in "silent" areas of white matter outnumber clinically apparent attacks by a factor of approximately five. No treatments have been convincingly shown to influence the course of primary progressive disease.

PSEUDOEXACERBATIONS

When we face an acute attack of MS, it is necessary to define as best we can what symptoms have appeared, how they affect the patient, and how long

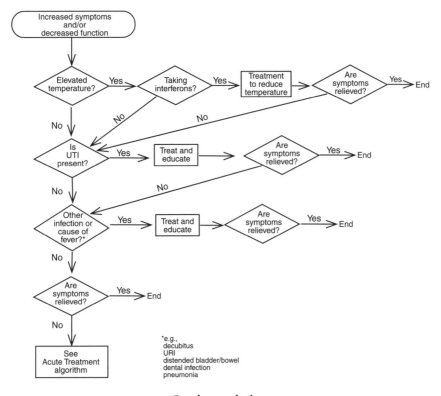

Pseudoexacerbations

they have been present. Major diagnostic considerations are the ability of infection to simulate an attack. People with MS are often extremely sensitive to small changes in body temperature. A minor febrile illness may reproduce old symptoms or produce new ones, and a low-grade fever may be incapacitating. It is essential to check for fever, to identify a source when fever is present, and to treat bacterial infection and reduce fever. Defervesence may eliminate the attack. Urinary tract infections are the most common offender, but common viral illnesses may also simulate attacks. Unusual environmental heat, such as the use of a Jacuzzi, may also precipitate a pseudoexacerbation.

TREATMENT OF EXACERBATIONS (RELAPSES)

If there is no infection or fever, the decision to be made is whether the attack merits treatment. If symptoms are mild and produce little functional deficit, it is reasonable to withhold treatment. There is some evidence

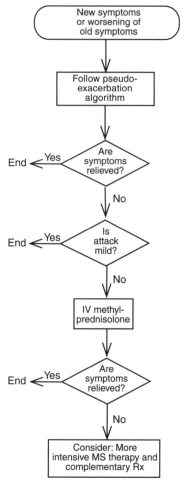

Acute Treatment

that although low-dose oral glucocorticoids may reduce symptoms, they may also predispose to subsequent relapses. In general, treat with high doses of glucocorticoids or not at all. A modest decline in acuity in one eye, minor diplopia, numbness in an arm or leg, or a sense of imbalance are examples of symptoms that might better be watched and not immediately treated.

Treatment should be undertaken if the attack is severe and produces a substantial impairment in areas such as vision, dexterity, ambulation, continence, coordination, perineal sensation, speech, or swallowing. The treatment of acute attacks has evolved over many years of empiricism without well-designed clinical trials. The most common practice is to use high-dose intravenous (IV) methyl prednisolone: 1000 mg in 100 to 250 ml normal saline given over 2 hours daily for 4 to 6 days. Some use 500 mg; some use 1500 mg; some use infusions at intervals of 2 or more days; some use infusions every 12 hours. It is common practice to follow this with a "taper" of oral prednisone over 2 to 6 weeks, beginning with 80 to 120 mg qd or qod and moving to progressively smaller doses every few days. The value of taper is uncertain and some physicians use IV steroids with abrupt cessation after a few days with no tapering.

Such courses are often repeated several times a year, based on the possible development of new symptoms. Some believe that a single infusion once a month has empiric benefit. There is some suggestion that the effects of oral steroids are comparable to those of intravenous administration, although most MS specialists prefer the IV route. Even larger doses of IV glucocorticoids are used in spinal cord injury. These large doses may help increase the amount of drug that will cross the blood–brain barrier and have an effect on lymphocyte function (see Chapter 1) that may last for weeks after the infusion.

Short courses of IV steroids are remarkably well tolerated and safe, with little evidence of long-term side effects. Short-term side effects include:

⊃ The infusions produce an unpleasant taste that may be helped by sucking on hard candy.

⊃ Induction of vascular headache is not uncommon.

⊃ Rarely, some patients have an urticarial hypersensitivity response requiring cessation of treatment.

⊃ Rapid infusion rates may trigger arrhythmias.

⊃ Diabetic patients may encounter severe grades of hyperglycemia; either infusions should be given with reduced frequency or an alternative regimen such as IV gamma globulin or plasmapheresis may be used. New antiinflammatory agents such as those that block adhesion molecule receptors on venular endothelial cells are being studied.

These treatments are usually given in outpatient settings or at home. After treatment, most patients feel energized and high, but the opposite effect may also be seen. Sleep is often disturbed for several days. A few patients become agitated, paranoid, or even psychotic for short periods of time; others slowly become more depressed.

For nonambulatory patients, some physicians prescribe subcutaneous low molecular weight or regular heparin every 12 hours. It is prudent to use an H_2 blocker such as ranitidine (Zantac®), 150 mg bid orally on infusion days; in one case, a perforated ulcer occurred on day 2 of infusions in a man with no history of dyspepsia. Use of a bedtime hypnotic for a few days is often helpful.

Improvement is often rapid and gratifying, but this same degree of improvement may also occur with no treatment. In some patients, a transient worsening of symptoms is seen before improvement. In some cases, there seems to be no effect. In attacks or first episodes of great severity, IV glucocorticoids may be followed with plasmapheresis, IV gamma globulin, and/or cyclophosphamide (Cytoxan®).

It is quite reasonable to use pulse glucocorticoids as defined previously when the diagnosis of MS is not proven but is the best working diagnosis. Consideration of long-term treatments does require a firm diagnosis.

TREATMENT TO ALTER THE DISEASE COURSE

With a firm diagnosis of relapsing-remitting MS, it is imperative that patients be informed about the three approved agents available for reducing attack rates and severity. Based on European and Canadian studies, it is likely that beta interferon is also helpful to prevent progression in secondary progressive disease (1). The three approved agents, beta interferon-1b (Betaseron®) (2), beta interferon-1a (Avonex®) (3,4,5), and glatiramer acetate (Copaxone®) (6), have been in use for several years to more than two decades. The clinical trials have been carefully performed, and all three agents have positive effects that are highly significant statistically and clinically. The safety of these agents is high. Unfortunately, the cost is also high—approximately $10,000 per year. However, in this context it should be noted that the average cost from care and loss of income in an impaired person with MS is at least $35,000 per year, economically supporting the use of these agents to reduce long-term disability.

Studies to compare the efficacy, safety, and complications of these treatments have not been done. There is no strong statistical evidence to support one of these agents over the others; there is some emerging sense that higher doses appear to be more effective.

Treatment needs to be sustained for years. It is commonly believed that the value of these agents is most evident after the first year or two of use. Their availability has for the first time offered a means to reduce MS-related disability. The disease is a lifelong process; without treatment a majority of patients will develop impairments in walking, cognition, and control of bladder and bowel function; fatigue; and/or poor balance. Changes are often subtle and may go unrecognized for long intervals. There are patients who have so-called "benign" MS, but with enough time and scrutiny the process often is not totally benign. For these reasons, we favor long-term treatment with these agents for most patients, with the

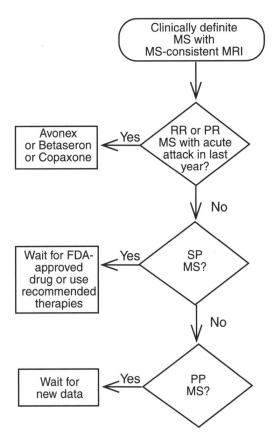

**Long-Term Treatment. RR = relapsing-remitting; PR = progressive-relapsing;
SP = secondary progressive; PP = primary progressive.**

exception of those with the primary progressive form. Treatment decisions require education, trust, and patience because side effects do occur, cost is high, and progression still occurs in many patients.

Beta interferon was developed in synthetic forms more than 10 years ago and was studied intensely for a possible role in the treatment of cancer. Natural interferon had minor effects in MS, and gamma interferon precipitated attacks and worsened MS manifestations. Beta interferon was thought to "downregulate" gamma interferon. The antiviral potential of beta interferon was also a theoretical consideration. It now appears that beta interferon reduces some aggressive elements of immune response such as gamma interferon, tumor necrosis factor, and other cytokines, while simultaneously promoting more gentle immunomodulatory cytokines such as interleukin-10.

Betaseron® (Berlex Laboratories)

Beta interferon-1b (Betaseron®) was the first of the three drugs to be approved, and it continues in active and growing use (1,2). Many patients have been receiving the drug for years and are advocates of its value. It is provided in the form of a powder that requires refrigeration. The vial contains 8 MIU or 0.25 mg of interferon, which is then reconstituted in diluent for subcutaneous injection every other day. Meticulous subcutaneous technique and rotation of sites needs to be taught. Ice before and after injection helps, as does massage of the injection site. Aloe vera juice or extract helps to reduce local reactions. Injection devices and needle-less bioinjectors are popular but expensive, and needle-free systems have not been tested for any possible impact on delivery of the drug. If another person can administer subcutaneous injections in the buttock, this site seems to be preferable. Serious skin reactions with localized necrosis occur in a small percentage of patients. If this happens more than once, it may be best to change to another agent.

When starting patients on beta interferon-1b, it is prudent to reduce the possibility of local and systemic reactions by using a fractional dose. Seventy-five percent of the dose is discarded for 1 to 5 weeks, then 50 percent is discarded for 3 to 6 weeks, then 25 percent is discarded for 2 to 6 weeks, then a full dose may be started. A few patients cannot tolerate the full dose and must remain at partial dosing permanently. Injections are usually administered every other day at bedtime.

Because interferons are responsible for much of the chills and fever experienced with viral illnesses, it is not surprising that their injection elicits the same response. These effects usually dissipate in 12 hours; as with any fever, disability may be transiently increased. Local and systemic side effects usually remit over a number of months. Curiously, local and systemic reactions may reappear and then disappear after months or years of treatment. Acetaminophen or acetylsalicylic acid given orally with the injection, and repeated several times, is often helpful. Ibuprofen also helps but is some times avoided because it has been shown to aggravate experimental allergic encephalomyelitis (EAE), an animal model for MS.

Avonex® (Biogen)

Beta interferon-1a (Avonex®) has also been approved for use in relapsing-remitting MS (3). Chemically, it is similar to beta interferon-1b but is glycosylated. It is given as an intramuscular injection of 0.03 mg (6 MIU) every 7 days. Local reactions are minor. Systemic reactions are significant at first but abate over time. Again, starting with a quarter- or half-dose and going to a full dose after a few weeks or months is often helpful. A dose of 10 mg of prednisone taken with the injection and again the morning after often helps at initiation. Refrigeration requirements for this drug are less stringent than those for Betaseron®. Because it is a weekly injection with few local reactions, it is more easily accepted by many patients. However, the dose is lower compared with Betaseron®, and some clinicians believe the benefit is also less.

Copaxone® (TevaMarion Partners)

Glatiramer acetate (Copaxone®) is very different from the interferons. More than 20 years ago this racemic mixture of peptides of glutamic acid, lysine, alanine, and tyrosine was shown to block EAE in animals. It has been widely used in Israel for years. It is injected as a 20 mg dose subcutaneously qd. Local reactions generally are mild. Systemic side effects are rare and usually insignificant. Carefully controlled U.S. trials have shown it to be safe and effective (6), and it is approved as an agent for relapsing-remitting MS. Study patients followed up for years have shown a suggested slowed rate of disease progression as well as a reduction in attack severity and frequency (6).

It is reasonable to consider these agents as equivalent for now. Betaseron has the most convincing data on reducing the disease burden on MRI, but injection site reactions and other side effects are limiting factors. Additionally, Betaseron induces neutralizing antibodies in some cases, which may reverse effectiveness, but the data are still unconvincing; if patients do poorly, switching to glatiramer acetate may be advised. Avonex® is generally well accepted by patients and is clearly effective, although some specialists believe that the dose is low. It also may induce neutralizing antibodies. It is probable that neutralizing antibodies to Avonex® will neutralize Betaseron® and vice versa. To date, there are no data to suggest that glatiramer loses its effect over time as a result of antibodies. The early studies on glatiramer acetate did not include sufficient MRI data, but new evidence shows benefit. There certainly are no present hard data to indicate that one of these agents is clearly superior to the others.

Trials of beta interferons-1a and -1b in secondary progressive disease in the United States will be completed in a year or two; based on positive European data, approval is expected. A trial of glatiramer acetate in primary progressive MS is under way. A form of beta interferon-1a marketed as Rebif®, which is chemically identical to Avonex®, has been used as a three times a week subcutaneous injection in Europe and Canada, at much higher doses than those for presently approved interferons in the United States. The results are impressive in both relapsing-remitting disease and secondary progressive disease, but as of the March 1999 Food and Drug

Administration review, Rebif was not approved for marketing until 2003, based on Orphan Drug Protection of Avonex®.

Monitoring laboratory data for glatiramer acetate is probably unnecessary. For the interferons, it is prudent to obtain semiannual liver panels and complete blood counts with differentials. Interferons may also induce hypertension.

Because a majority of people with MS are women in their childbearing years, the potential risk of these three agents needs to be carefully considered. The natural immunomodulation of pregnancy to permit the presence of foreign DNA seems to have an ameliorative effect on MS, but postpartum flares are common. The potential teratogenic effects of these drugs is not known, although animal studies indicate that the risk is small. Interferons may trigger spontaneous abortion in animals.

The manufacturers of these agents urge that the drugs be used only with adequate contraception. This poses a problem for young women with MS, who must consider postponement of therapy until planned pregnancies have been completed. Women who want to have children and whose probability of achieving pregnancy may require months or years should consider the risks of these agents and incorporate this into their decision-making process. They should discontinue treatment when pregnancy is confirmed. Breast-feeding poses another problem. One approach is bottle-feeding; another is the use of once-weekly Avonex with breast pumping and discarding of milk for 24 hours after injection. There are no good data on the potential risks, but the risks of postponing these treatments for years into the future is certainly known.

Various empiric steps should be undertaken in patients who continue to show serious progression while receiving these agents; these steps include the addition of intermittent infusions of methylprednisolone; weekly oral or injected methotrexate (7); daily azathioprine; monthly IV gamma globulin; and various chemotherapeutic regimens such as cyclophosphamide, cladribine, and mitoxantrone. These regimens are difficult to manage and should be undertaken by neurologists who are familiar with their use in MS. Some patients with substantial financial means and a tolerance for injections combine interferon with glatiramer. It should be noted that all of these combination drug approaches are anecdotal, uncontrolled, and unconfirmed. The nature of our health care system makes controlled comparative and combined trials difficult to support.

SUMMARY

Once a diagnosis of MS has been made, it is necessary to deal with long-term management issues, including the management of symptoms, the management of acute attacks, and the use of recently developed therapies to minimize disease progression. Symptoms associated with the disease affect wellness, independence, careers, and families, and the establishment of trusting and supportive relationships within which these issues can be addressed is essential.

REFERENCES

1. Knight R, Hern J, Coleman R, et al. for the European study group on interferon beta-1b in secondary progressive MS. Placebo-controlled multicentre randomised trial of interferon beta-1b in treatment of secondary progressive multiple sclerosis. *Lancet* 1998; 352:1491–1497.
2. The IFNB MS study group. Interferon beta-1B in the treatment of multiple sclerosis. *Neurology* 1995; 45:1277–1285.7
3. Jacobs LD, Cookfair DL, et al. for the MSCRG. Intramuscular interferon beta 1-a for disease progression in relapsing multiple sclerosis. *Ann Neurol* 1996; 39:285–294.
4. PRISMS study group. Randomised double-blind placebo controlled study of interferon beta 1-a in relapsing-remitting multiple sclerosis. *Lancet* 1998; 352:1498–1504.
5. Li D, Guojun Z, Hyde R, et al. Comparison of the therapeutic effect of interferon beta 1-a on baseline MRI activity. *J Neurol* 1998; 245:385–386.
6. Johnson, KP, Brooks BR, et al. for the copolymer 1 MS study group. Extended use of glatiramer acetate is well tolerated and maintains its clinical effect on MS relapse rate and degree of disability. *Neurology* 1996; 50:701–708.
7. Goodkin DE, Rudick RA, VanderBrug Medendorp S, et al. Low dose methotrexate reduces the rate of progression in chronic progressive multiple sclerosis. *Ann Neurol* 1995; 37:30–40.

CHAPTER 3

Fatigue

Randall T. Schapiro, MD,
and Diana M. Schneider, PhD

Of the broad constellation of symptoms that occur in multiple sclerosis (MS), fatigue is one of the most common and often the most disabling. Fatigue is reported by more than 50 percent of all individuals with MS as one of their worst problems (1,2,3), and it is a major cause of unemployment in people with MS. Krupp (3) notes that people with MS generally describe fatigue as "an overwhelming sense of tiredness, lack or energy, or feeling of exhaustion." The Panel on Fatigue of the Multiple Sclerosis Council for Clinical Practice Guidelines (4) defined fatigue as "a subjective lack of physical and/or mental energy that is perceived by the individual or caregiver to interfere with usual and desired activities."

Before fatigue can be managed, its causes must be identified, and may be found singly or intermixed in various combinations at any time.

⊃ People with MS experience normal fatigue, but there is a natural tendency to attribute all problems to the disease itself.

⊃ People with MS often require a large expenditure of effort to accomplish a limited objective; for example, walking up or down stairs may consume an amount of energy well beyond that used by a person without MS. This excessive energy use produces early or premature fatigue.

⊃ A person with MS may become deconditioned for various reasons.

⊃ Fatigue secondary to depression, both exogenous and endogenous, is common in MS.

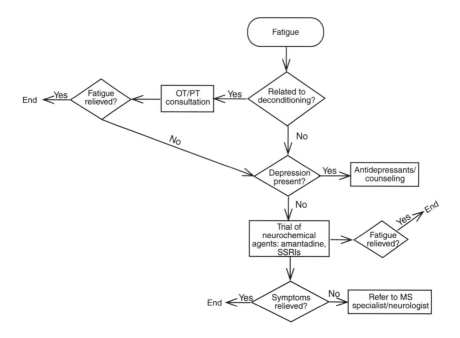

Fatigue

○ Fatigue may also result from taking a number of medications commonly used to treat the symptoms of MS and other conditions, including certain analgesics, anticonvulsants, antidepressants, antihistamines, antihypertensive agents, antiinflammatory agents, and many others.

○ People with MS commonly experience a "short-circuiting" type of fatigue that is a direct result of demyelination.

When we speak of fatigue in MS, however, we are most often referring to the debilitating "MS fatigue" that may also be described as "idiopathic lassitude" (5). It is this type of fatigue that presents the greatest problem in MS and is the least amenable to treatment. It presents as a generalized, rapidly induced tiredness that patients describe as "coming out of nowhere" and often describe as similar to the feeling of exhaustion that accompanies the "flu."

This type of fatigue can be distinguished from the fatigue associated with depression, limb weakness, and sleepiness (3,6). It comes on easily, without warning, prevents sustained physical functioning, is worsened by heat, and makes it difficult to work productively; it is a major reason many people with MS are forced to cease working. MS fatigue may appear quite early in the disease, frequently in the absence of severe neurologic involvement. Indeed, there appears to be little correlation of the Expanded Disability Status Score (EDSS) with the extent of fatigue; some people with relatively mild disease are seriously incapacitated by fatigue, whereas others with significant disability have little fatigue. Sleepiness often accompanies this type of fatigue even if the person has had a good night's sleep. A short nap may be therapeutic. A tepid bath or a period of spa exercise in warm but not hot water may also help.

Most people who experience MS-related fatigue are sensitive to heat and tend to do better in cooler climates and in winter rather than summer. Fatigue often worsens during the day, often being most disabling in the afternoon, corresponding to peak body temperature.

It is impossible to separate the management of fatigue from that of numerous other symptoms of the disease, especially weakness and spasticity (7), but also including pain, poor sleep, psychological stress, and deconditioning (3). In turn, fatigue itself contributes to a worsening of these and other symptoms of MS.

In addition to affecting motor-related symptoms, MS fatigue affects the ability of many patients to work efficiently on cognitive functions such as reading and to absorb complex information. When they are experiencing fatigue, MS patients have prolonged reaction times compared with periods when they are experiencing less fatigue (8,9). These studies suggest that both attention and memory are affected by fatigue. A sudden increase in fatigue may also be a sign of an impending relapse, especially if it is accompanied by new neurologic symptoms or signs (3).

PHARMACOLOGIC MANAGEMENT

Amantadine is an antiviral agent that is also a dopamine agonist. It has been widely used to treat fatigue in MS, although its mechanism of action is not known. A number of clinical trials have shown substantial improvement in one or more factors used to measure fatigue (10,11,12). It is generally given in a dose of 100 mg two times a day.

Side effects generally are mild and infrequent but may include hallucinations, vivid dreams, nausea, hyperactivity, anxiety, insomnia, constipation, and rash. Few people discontinue the medication as a result of side effects. Approximately one third of patients regard this drug as valuable.

Many patients who have fatigue that does not respond to amantadine will respond to relatively low doses of fluoxetine (Prozac®), whether they have depressive symptoms or not.

In the authors' experience, pemoline (Cylert®), a CNS stimulant that has also been used to treat fatigue associated with MS (12,13), is most effective for fatigue that tends to occur at a specific time of day. Long-term treatment has not been well studied, but the drug is often effective in the short term at a dose of 37.5–75 mg per day. Both amantadine and pemoline may be used intermittently. Recent warnings regarding pemoline should be addressed: obtain baseline liver function evaluation before use and periodically thereafter, and advise patients to report symptoms of liver involvement, such as nausea, anorexia, or jaundice.

Patients who do appear to have depressive symptoms coexisting with fatigue should be evaluated for clinical depression, with appropriate pharmacologic therapy or psychiatric referral as appears appropriate. If pharmacologic therapy is elected, it is preferable to choose those antidepressants that are least sedating, such as fluoxetine (Prozac®), sertraline (Zoloft®), or bupropion (Wellbutin®).

NONPHARMACOLOGIC THERAPIES

Some patients with MS respond well to a carefully designed program of aerobic exercise. Although people with MS may have been told to limit such exercise because of the increase in fatigue that results from any increase in body temperature, it has now been demonstrated that they can improve fitness (14,15). It is becoming increasingly clear that people with MS can and should participate in regular exercise. Swimming is of particular benefit because it does not result in an increase of core body temperature.

Many MS patients report a substantial reduction in fatigue from cooling therapy using either active or passive cooling garments. Few scientific data are as yet available demonstrating the effectiveness of this type of therapy. The garments are often quite expensive and cumbersome to use.

A personalized strategy to conserve energy is a good way to manage MS fatigue (5). Occupational therapists are helpful in teaching concepts of energy conservation to those who have moderate or severe fatigue. Efficiency in performing activities of daily living, including dressing, grooming, toileting, and eating, may increase the energy available for other activities (16).

To enable patients to maximize energy and minimize overexertion, Schapiro and colleagues (17) recommend that patients:

⊃ Sleep regular hours and avoid unnecessary late nights.

⊃ Plan ahead and make daily or weekly schedules of activities.

⊃ Recognize their limits, which may vary from day to day.

⊃ Pace their activities, taking short rest periods during prolonged activity.

A period of rest of 10 to 15 minutes several times a day is restorative and may substitute for more prolonged periods of rest that may include sleep (15).

SUMMARY

The management of fatigue in MS requires understanding, proper diagnosis, and appropriate management. The strategies are based on the type of fatigue, along with the common-sense tools of energy conservation as taught by occupational therapists.

REFERENCES

1. Fisk JD, Pontefract A, Ritvo PG, et al. The impact of fatigue on patients with MS. *Can J Neurol Sci* 1994; 21:9–14.
2. Krupp LB. Mechanisms, measurement, and management of fatigue in multiple sclerosis. In: Thompson AJ, Polman C, Hohlfeld R (eds.). *Multiple sclerosis: Clinical challenges and controversies*. London: Martin Dunitz, 1997:283–291.
3. Krupp LB, Elkins LE. Management of fatigue in multiple sclerosis. In: Burks JS, Johnson KP (eds.). *Multiple sclerosis: Diagnosis, medical management, and rehabilitation*. New York: Demos, 2000 (In Press).
4. Multiple Sclerosis Council for Clinical Practice Guidelines. "Fatigue and Multiple Sclerosis: Evidence-Based Management Strategies for Fatigue in Multiple Sclerosis," 1998, Paralyzed Veterans of America.
5. Schapiro RT. *Symptom management in multiple sclerosis*, 3rd ed. New York: Demos, 1998.
6. Krupp LB, Alvarez LA, LaRocca NG, et al. Fatigue in multiple sclerosis. *Arch Neurol* 1998; 45: 435–437.
7. Schapiro RT, Schneider DS. *Symptom management in multiple sclerosis*. In: Halper J, Holland NJ (eds.). *Comprehensive nursing care in multiple sclerosis*. New York: Demos, 1997:25–44.
8. Sandroni P, Walker C, Starr A. Fatigue in patients with MS. *Arch Neurol* 1992; 49:517–524.
9. Elkins LE, Pollina DA, Scheffer SR, Krupp LB. Effects of fatigue on cognitive functioning in multiple sclerosis. *Neurology* 1998; 50(S):A126.

10. Canadian MS Research Group. A randomized controlled trial of amantadine in fatigue associated with multiple sclerosis. *Can J Neurol Sci* 1987; 14:273–278.
11. Cohen RA, Fisher M. Amantadine treatment of fatigue associated with MS. *Arch Neurol* 1989; 46:676–680.
12. Krupp LB, Coyle PK, Doscher C, et al. Fatigue therapy in MS: Results of a double-blind, randomized, parallel trial of amantadine, pemoline, and placebo. *Neurology* 1995; 45:1956–1961.
13. Weinshenker BG, Penman M, Bass B, et al. A double-blind, randomized, crossover trial of pemoline in fatigue associated with multiple sclerosis. *Neurology* 1992; 42:1468–1471.
14. Petajan JH, Gappmaier E, White AT, et al. Impact of aerobic training on fitness and quality of life in multiple sclerosis. *Ann Neurol* 1996; 39:432–431.
15. Petajan JH. Weakness. In: Burks JS, Johnson KP (eds.). *Multiple sclerosis: Diagnosis, medical management, and rehabilitation.* New York: Demos, 2000 (In Press).
16. Wolf BG. Occupational therapy for patients with multiple sclerosis. In: Maloney FP, Burks JS, Ringel SP (eds.). *Interdisciplinary rehabilitation of multiple sclerosis and neuromuscular disorders.* Philadelphia: JB Lippincott, 1985:103–128.
17. Schapiro RT, Baumhefner RW, Tourtellotte WW. Multiple sclerosis: A clinical viewpoint to management. In: Raine CS, McFarland HF, Tourtellotte WW (eds.). *Multiple sclerosis: Clinical and pathogenetic basis.* London: Chapman & Hall, 1997:391–420.

CHAPTER 4

Spasticity, Balance, Tremor, and Weakness: Factors in Mobility Impairment

Randall T. Schapiro, MD,
and Diana M. Schneider, PhD

Multiple sclerosis (MS) frequently results in impaired movement. Despite its relatively low incidence, MS was the second most common condition linked with activity limitation in the period from 1990 to 1992 (1); 69.4 percent of the 180,000 individuals with MS who participated in this survey complained of limited activity.

The major symptoms that affect mobility are spasticity, balance and coordination difficulties, tremor, and weakness. These symptoms can be disabling individually or in combination. A vicious cycle may be established when weakness—due to corticospinal tract involvement, fatigue, depression, and/or heat intolerance—leads to reduced exercise and resultant disuse atrophy, contracture, and deconditioning (2). Every symptom that affects mobility has the power to affect quality of life; each requires management strategies to minimize disability and maximize the ability to lead a normal life.

SPASTICITY

Spasticity is generally a component of spastic paresis and is defined as a velocity-dependent increased resistance of muscle to stretch due to activation of tonic stretch reflexes (3). Patients with MS most often experience *spinal* spasticity, in which the limbs are flexed and adducted and exaggerated responses to cutaneous stimulation are present (4). Spasticity occurs most frequently in the muscles that are responsible for maintaining upright posture. In the lower limbs, the muscle groups most likely to develop spasticity and be at risk for contractures are the iliopsoas, the quadriceps, the hamstrings, and the gastrocnemius (2). A small amount of spasticity does not have a significant effect on function, but when it becomes more prominent it can hamper gait, seating, and comfort. Spasticity may become extremely painful.

Spasticity is not always a disadvantage; stiff muscles can provide support for the patient's body against gravity when walking, thus permitting greater mobility. However, rapid or highly coordinated movements are no longer possible because the individual can no longer modulate muscle activity to suit momentary changes in the environment (4).

Increased stiffness in the muscles may mean that a great amount of energy is required to perform everyday activities. Reducing spasticity can produce greater freedom of movement and strength, frequently accompanied by less fatigue and increased coordination. Optimal management must include classic rehabilitation techniques to maximize the use of existing function and to prevent secondary manifestations such as clonus. The major means to reduce spasticity include stretching, range of motion exercise, and a variety of medications. When spasticity is severe, surgery may be necessary.

Painful flexor spasms and increased muscle tone are also an aspect of impaired motor control; they may be produced by any increase in nociceptive input, including urinary tract infection, constipation, pressure sores, ingrown toenails, or broken bones, or by some antidepressants and interferon beta-1b (4). Attention to such factors may significantly reduce spasticity.

The simplest way to reduce spasticity is *passive stretching*, in which each affected joint is slowly moved into a position that stretches the spastic muscles. Once the muscles reach their stretched position, they are held there for approximately 1 minute to allow slow relaxation and release undesired tension. This stretching program begins at the ankle to stretch the calf muscles, then proceeds to the muscles in the back of the thigh, the buttocks, the groin, and, after turning from back to stomach, the muscles on the front of the thigh. Spending some time each day in the prone position may relax the shoulder muscles, which otherwise predispose to flexion.

Attention to range of motion is key to maintaining mobility and skin integrity (2). Range of motion exercises differ from stretching exercises in that the movement about the joint is not held for any specific length of time. Both passive stretching and range of motion exercises are commonly taught by a physical therapist who is experienced with MS.

Exercising in a pool or spa may also be beneficial because the buoyancy of water allows movements to be performed with less energy expen-

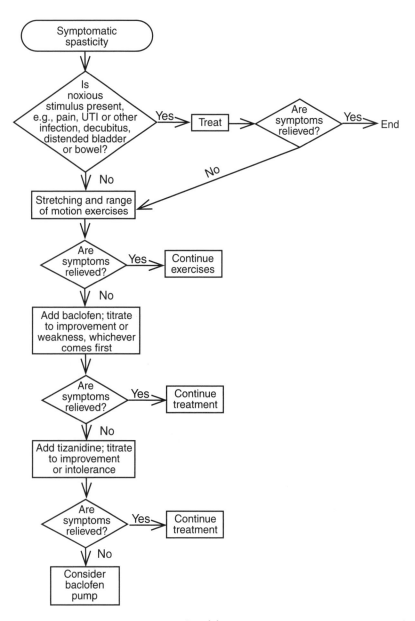

Spasticity

diture, facilitating both stretching and range of motion exercises. These exercises consist of easy, slow, rhythmic, and flowing calisthenics that allow most of the joints to move through their full stretching range. The water temperature should be cool to lukewarm, approximately 80–84°; warmer temperatures should be avoided because significant fatigue may result.

Spasticity may also be reduced by relaxation techniques that involve a combination of progressive tensing and relaxing of individual muscles, accompanied by deep breathing techniques and imagery.

Mechanical Aids

Specific devices can counteract spasticity and prevent contractures. For example, a "toe spreader" or "finger spreader" can be used to relax tightness in the feet and hands and to aid mobility. Orthoses for the wrist, foot, and hand can be made to maintain a natural position and prevent limitations on movement and deformities. For example, an ankle-foot orthosis can be made to place the foot at many different angles to the ankle. A good orthotist can make the brace to take stress off the knee. Hinges in the material can add to its flexibility. All orthoses should be customized to allow for maximal benefit.

Medications

Baclofen (Lioresal®) is the most common antispasticity drug used in MS, and most patients respond well to it. The dose must be carefully determined for each individual; too little will be ineffective, whereas too much produces fatigue and a feeling of weakness. The correct dose is usually determined by starting at a low level and slowly increasing the amount until a maximum beneficial effect is achieved. The most common error when taking baclofen is to give up on it before it has reached the dose necessary to obtain proper relaxation. That dose may be as low as 5 mg per day, but as much as 40 mg four times a day may be necessary.

Tizanidine (Zanaflex®) has effects on spasticity that are similar to those of baclofen. It produces greater sedation than baclofen but less weakness, and may therefore be a useful medication for those in whom sedation is less of a concern than weakness. It may also be used in combination with baclofen, particularly as a nighttime dose when sedation may be a positive feature. The dose should be kept to the minimum needed for benefit in order to minimize sedation (4).

Another drug that sometimes is helpful in relieving spasticity is sodium dantrolene (Dantrium®), which acts directly on the muscle. It can be helpful, but it may induce weakness—even at low doses—and may cause liver toxicity. Spasticity may also be reduced by diazepam (Valium®), which is most often used at night because its calming effect also helps to induce sleep. Its strong sedative effect limits its use during the daytime. Clonazepam (Klonopin®) is closely related to diazepam. Its main use has been to treat certain types of epilepsy. It produces significant relaxation and thus may be used as an antispasticity medication. Like diazepam, it sedates and is therefore best used at night. When using diazepam or clonazepam, both the physician and the person with MS must keep in mind the potential for chemical dependency. Lorazepam (Ativan®) is also effective.

Another drug commonly used for back spasms is cyclobenzaprine hydrochloride (Flexeril®), which acts quite specifically on such spasms, but may settle limb spasms as well. It usually works best in combination with another spasticity medication, but it is very sedating in many patients. Any of these drugs may become less effective when taken for a prolonged period, requiring cessation for a period of time, after which they may again become effective. Some data suggest that gabapentin (Neurontin®) may reduce spasticity in doses of 300–900 mg every 8 hours.

People with MS occasionally develop "paroxysmal" or "tonic" spasms, in which a limb may assume the flexor or extensor position. Carbamazepine (Tegretol®) generally controls such spasms, although baclofen may also be effective. Cortisone may decrease spasticity in general and is effective for paroxysmal spasms when used on a short-term basis; its long-term use is not advocated because of numerous risks.

Another approach to the management of severe spasticity involves the use of a pump to deliver baclofen intrathecally. A tube is placed in the spinal canal and connected underneath the skin to the pump in the abdominal region, through which the drug is delivered intrathecally. The newest pumps can be programmed by computer via radio waves so that the dose can be changed as needed. For some patients, this technique may provide relief of intractable spasticity. Because the required doses of baclofen are so low (micrograms), side effects are also low and there is almost always a significant decrease in fatigue and malaise. This technique may be especially useful with nonambulatory patients; severe spasticity may be transformed into flaccid paresis, which makes daily function and nursing care much easier. This treatment is aggressive and expensive. It should be reserved for those with severe spasticity that cannot be adequately managed by oral medications.

Surgical Management

Spasms occasionally become so severe that no medication is effective. When this occurs, a phenol motor point block may be indicated. This produces decreased tone in the muscles, which may be more comfortable but usually does not increase functional mobility.

Local injections of botulinum toxin (Botox®), which blocks release of acetylcholine from motor nerve endings, are effective in weakening any muscle for approximately 3 months (5). Botulinum toxin causes a temporary blockage within the muscle; it is somewhat easier to control than phenol but may need more repetitive injections. This treatment is practical for small muscle spasms, especially around the eye or face. Severe spasms may be managed by surgical procedures that involve cutting nerves or tendons to decrease the contraction of specific muscles that are producing serious stiffness.

The faithful use of an exercise program and the appropriate use of drugs when needed significantly increase the level of function and avoid the development of these more severe problems.

TREMOR

Tremor is one of the most frustrating symptoms to treat in MS and can be a major cause of diminished function. There are many different kinds of tremors; some have gross oscillations, others are fine; some occur at rest, others occur only with purposeful movement; some are fast, others are slow; some affect the limbs, others may involve the head, trunk, or speech; some are disabling, others are merely a nuisance; and some are treatable, others are not. As with all symptoms, because of this wide variation, proper diagnosis is essential before correct management decisions can be made.

Pharmacologic Management

The most common tremor seen in MS—and the most difficult to treat—occurs as the result of demyelination in the cerebellum and its pathways, which often results in a gross tremor that is relatively slow and occurs with purposeful movement of the arm or leg. This type of tremor is almost always exaggerated during times of stress and anxiety, so one mode of managing the problem is treatment with drugs that have a calming or sedative effect. Hydroxyzine (Atarax® and Vistaril®) is an antihistamine that may settle a minor tremor that has been magnified by stress. Clonazepam (Klonopin®) may also decrease a tremor via its sedative effect. The antitremor effect must be balanced against the generally unwanted effects of sedation by carefully monitoring the dose until the desired effect is achieved. Propranolol (Inderal®) and INH (isoniazid) have been used historically to treat tremor but with disappointing results. The long-acting preparations of propranolol have a smoother and more salutary effect (e.g., propranolol LA 60 mg one or more times a day).

Some studies have shown that low doses (50–200 mg three times a day) of the anticonvulsant primidone (Mysoline®) may alleviate this difficult symptom, although it is sedating. Low doses may be worthwhile. Acetazolamide (Diamox®) is a diuretic that has some antitremor properties and may be of value in selected patients.

Because a component of spasm is often involved in gross tremors, baclofen may provide some relief. The potential but reversible side effect of weakness must be balanced against the tremor-reducing effect of the drug, again by careful adjustment of the dose.

Recent studies indicate a reasonable response to the anti-anxiety drug buspirone (Buspar®), which is nonsedating and nonaddictive.

Other Treatments for the Management of Tremor

Drugs are not the complete solution to the management of tremor. Physical techniques provide another approach. Physical treatments fall into three general categories:

Patterning is a controversial technique that is used by physical and occupational therapists to trace and repeat basic movement patterns. It is based on the theory that certain muscles can be trained to move in a coordinated fashion by repeatedly using the nervous circuit involved in a movement. These normal movements are guided and assisted by the therapist until they become automatic. Minor resistance is then added and removed while the patient repeats the patterns independently. The muscles gradually appear to develop increased endurance for these learned movements and manage to retain control when the patterns are applied to functional tasks.

Immobilization is the placement of a rigid brace across a joint, fixing it in one position and dampening the severity of a tremor by reducing random movement in the joint. Bracing is most helpful in the ankle and foot, providing a stable base for standing and walking. It may also be used for the arm and hand. The desired position of function is defined by the tasks that are to be facilitated, such as writing, eating, or knitting; the brace is used to immobilize the arm or hand for these tasks and then removed. Lightweight high-top shoes with leather soles may be helpful.

Weighting involves the addition of weight to a part of the body to provide increased control over its movements. The underlying theory behind this approach is that more muscles will be used to stabilize a distant point in the body (hands, wrists, feet, ankles) when a heavier object is involved. This stabilizing action tends to reduce tremor and provide greater sensory feedback to the brain. In practical terms, either the limb itself may be weighted or the object being used may be made heavier, including utensils, pens and pencils, canes, or walkers.

These techniques are used primarily for tremors that affect the limbs. Their goal is to teach the person with MS to compensate for tremor by providing as much stability for the limbs as possible. It may be important to develop postural adjustments, such as using one's arms close to the body. Adaptive equipment and/or assistive devices that are nonskid, easy to grasp, and stable are helpful and can be used for many activities.

Tremors of the head, neck, and upper torso are more difficult to manage than those of the limbs. Stabilizing the neck with a brace may be helpful.

Stereotactic surgery has occasionally been used to control cerebellar tremor, but results are mixed and this procedure is generally used only as a last resort (6). Deep brain stimulation and thalamic stimulation are currently being explored as possible means to reduce MS tremor.

Tremors of the lips, tongue, or jaw may affect speech by interfering either with breath control for phrasing and loudness or with the ability to form and pronounce sounds. Speech therapy may involve changing the rate of speaking or the phrasing of sentences. Suggestions may be made as to the placement of the lips, tongue, or jaw for the best possible sound production. A simple pace board—a pattern of rectangles set next to each other—may slow the person down and allow for improved understanding. The person points to each square while uttering a single syllable. If he or she can slow down to keep pace with the pointing, a dramatic increase in clarity of speech often results. Pace boards can be simple and effective at virtually no cost. In some instances, tremor may make it impossible to speak, in which case alternative communication devices must be used.

Oscillating movements of the eyes (oscillopsia) are a severe source of disability for some patients. Large does of gabapentin (Neurontin®) may be helpful. Adjusting head position to reduce tremor is also helpful. Covering one eye with an opaque lens may also reduce symptoms.

None of these techniques completely eliminates the problem of tremor. The goal is continued function, which can often be achieved by combining some of these therapies.

BALANCE AND COORDINATION

Vertigo, imbalance, and incoordination are frequent problems in MS. They put individuals at risk for falls and injury, which complicates management and increases disability. A fall with a fracture is a common event that will move a patient from being ambulatory with a cane or a walker to permanent wheelchair status (6).

Control of balance is complex and involves essentially every part of the nervous system. For this reason, lesions in a number of areas may affect the

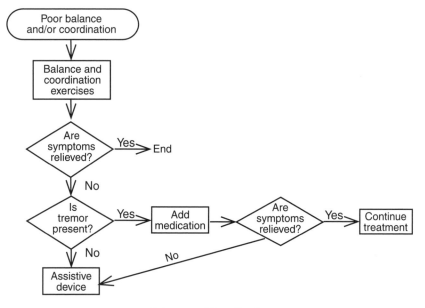

Balance and Coordination

MS patient's balance and coordination. These include the visual system, proprioceptive system, vestibular system, and sensorimotor system. Cerebellar incoordination and tremor are among the most difficult MS symptoms to treat and often are incapacitating (6).

An aid to enhance ambulatory mobility becomes essential if balance or coordination is a problem. Whether a cane, crutch, or walker is used, it is necessary that it be correctly sized and properly used. This is best accomplished by a skilled physical therapist. The advent of new large-wheel walkers with hand controls, a seat, and a basket has been a significant innovation for many patients.

WEAKNESS

Weakness is experienced by at least half of all people who have MS. Ambulatory patients who walk a short distance may begin with no symptoms of weakness, only to develop a limp and progressive weakness so that walking becomes impossible. In some instances, weakness is a symptom of a developing exacerbation; when this occurs, weakness is the symptom least likely to recover completely (7).

It is vital that the source of weakness be understood in order to properly manage it; if it is due to deconditioning, weakness may be improved by

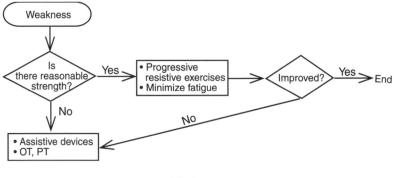

Weakness

lifting weights (progressive resistive exercise). Specifically, progressive resistive exercises targeting the disused muscles may be helpful. However, when weakness is due to poor nerve conduction in the spinal cord and the brain, excessive exercise may add to the fatigue.

Physical therapy is integral to the management of weakness in MS. To enhance function, the physical therapist attempts to substitute the use of uninvolved muscles for those whose function is impaired. As noted by Brar and Wangaard (8), frequently used techniques include:

⊃ active assistive exercise and active exercises

⊃ proprioceptive neuromuscular facilitation (PNF) technique

⊃ therapeutic exercises

⊃ resistive exercises

It is impossible to separate the management of weakness from that of spasticity and fatigue. If muscles are less stiff, less energy needs to be expended in movement. Medications or other treatments that lessen spasticity also increase strength. Similarly, lessening fatigue may also increase strength.

Efficiency is the key to increasing strength in patients with MS. Energy should be conserved and wisely used. This means using one's muscles for practical, enjoyable activities and planning the use of time accordingly; difficult activities should be done before those that are easier to perform. Assistive devices may also be helpful in increasing overall efficiency.

Aerobic exercise is possible for MS patients and results in a significant improvement in both aerobic capacity and muscle strength (7). Strength may be increased by using an aerobic exercise machine such as an exercycle or a rowing machine. The principle of not becoming fatigued and exercising those muscles that can be strengthened to compensate for the weaker muscles must be applied.

Because a substantial percentage of MS patients are sensitive to heat, exercise that increases core body temperature has the capacity to increase weakness. For this reason, exercising in an air-conditioned room or a pool is highly recommended. It is important that the person with MS be adequately hydrated, especially during exercise. Many patients refrain from drinking, especially before or during social occasions, because of poor bladder control (see Chapter 6). Dehydration is thus a common problem; it reduces the circulating blood volume, which in turn enhances fatigue (7).

As with other symptoms of MS, weakness may mimic other disorders, including stroke, root compression involving radiculopathy, and movement disorders. It is important, however, not to dismiss the possibility that such conditions may be coexistent with MS without appropriate testing. Among the disorders whose symptoms may mimic MS are Bell's palsy, radiculopathy, neuropathy and "pseudoneuropathy," stroke, myasthenia gravis, and myopathic disorders that produce proximal weakness such as polymyositis (7). Metastatic bone disease with cord compression can also mimic MS weakness.

AMBULATION

Mobility impairment is frequently associated with MS. Approximately 65 percent of patients are able to walk 25 years after diagnosis (9); how well and frequently they walk—and how well they are able to function in the community—is closely linked to careful management of the symptoms discussed in the preceding section.

If ambulation becomes impaired, a more practical means to accomplish this goal should be substituted. Emotional consequences must be addressed because people value being ambulatory far beyond its true value.

"Foot drop" is manifested when the toes of the affected foot touch the ground before the heel, disrupting balance and causing falls. A polypropylene insert used inside the shoe to keep the foot from dropping is very effective. This lightweight ankle-foot orthosis—or AFO—picks up the foot and allows it to follow through in the normal heel-foot manner. Ankle-foot orthoses can also be designed to decrease spasticity by tilting the foot to a specified angle and keeping it from inverting or everting. The proper use of an AFO decreases fatigue while increasing stability.

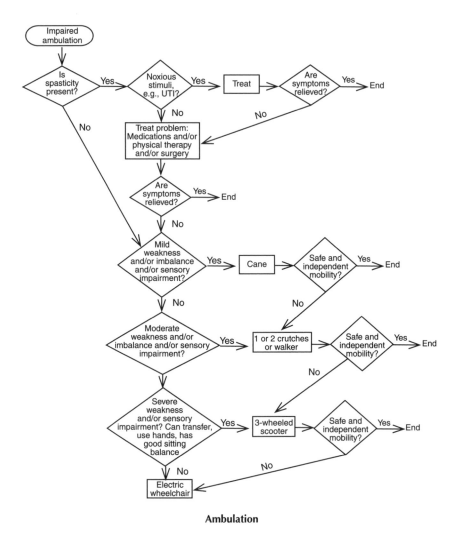

Ambulation

If the hip muscles are also weak, the leg will swing out in front to allow the foot to clear the ground. In order to maintain stability, the knee is often forced into hyperextension, which puts significant stress on the knee. After a period of time, the knee begins to hurt and may become swollen secondary to arthritis. To prevent this condition, a metal device called a Swedish hyperextension cage can prevent the knee from snapping back. Alternatively, a custom-made knee brace may be necessary.

If balance is also a problem, an assistive device such as a cane may be needed. Two canes may be needed if weakness is pronounced in both legs.

If balance and weakness are more severe, it may be necessary to use fore-arm Lofstrand crutches. These crutches provide greater stability than a cane, and their use does not require as much strength in the upper extremities. Walkers are important aids, and the newer style large-wheel walkers with hand controls, a basket, and a seat are a boon for many patients.

If walking is still difficult or impossible, a wheelchair may be the correct choice. Ultra-lightweight wheelchairs are often helpful in patients with well-preserved arm strength, but they may add to fatigue. A three-wheeled motorized scooter can be a boon for people with MS because it does not carry the stigma associated with a standard wheelchair. A motorized scooter is best used by those who have retained some means of walking because the seating system is not designed for all-day sitting. Adequate sitting balance and the use of the upper extremities are also essential.

Those who do not possess the skills necessary to use a three-wheeler appropriately may achieve independence using a lightweight motorized wheelchair. A standard manual wheelchair often does not offer sufficient independence because of the fatigue generated by operating the chair and the coordination necessary to control it. The key in choosing a chair or scooter is *independence*. The proper device should be selected to regain control and independence in the environment. Help from a physical therapist or a physiatrist is necessary to select the most appropriate mobility device.

PREVENTING IMMOBILITY

People with MS are too often told to rest and not overdo, and the fear of fatigue becomes almost unbearable. There is no real basis for this fear. *People with MS are not fragile!* Proper exercise leads to increased fitness and less fatigue. The process is slow, and it begins with a carefully developed exercise prescription. Like medicine, exercise should be prescribed by a professional—usually a physical therapist or a physician—who knows how to tailor the exercises to the individual. The exercise prescription should have four elements:

1. The type of exercise (aerobic, strengthening, balance, stretching)
2. The duration of exercise (how long to exercise)
3. The frequency of exercise (how often to exercise)
4. The intensity of exercise (how hard to exercise)

The role of exercise in MS has become somewhat controversial, partly because the meaning of exercise is misunderstood. To many, exercise is defined as stressing one's body to the point of pain, an approach whose watchwords are "no pain, no gain." But in MS it has become quite clear that if one exercises to the point of pain, fatigue sets in and weakness increases.

Rigorous exercise also increases core body temperature. Because myelin has been damaged or destroyed, this rise in temperature further increases weakness. Thus, it is fairly obvious why exercise originally fell into bad repute with those knowledgeable about MS.

Our understanding of what is "good" exercise for people with MS and how they should train has increased considerably in the past few years as the concept of fitness has developed. Fitness implies general overall health. It is a holistic concept that strives for improvement in function of the heart, lungs, muscles, and other organs, and is attained by adhering to a proper diet, not smoking, and exercising appropriately.

Two major concepts underlie the term *appropriate*. First, because of the wide variability of the disease, what is "good" exercise for one person may not be good for another. *It is important to tailor an exercise program for each individual rather than to have a set program for everyone who has MS.* The second factor is that there are many kinds of exercise—not just those that involve running, jumping, or similar activities.

Exercises that increase mobility through stretching and maintaining range of motion play an important part in combating weakness by reducing the stiffness so commonly present in MS. Relaxation exercises are particularly helpful in reducing stress, which can increase weakness and fatigue; techniques for learning how to relax must be considered as part of any overall program designed to reduce weakness and fatigue.

Moderate aerobic exercises, which may involve a stationary bicycle, rowing machine, treadmill (one that stops when the runner does), brisk walking, running, or a self-wheel in a wheelchair, will result in a slow but definite increase in endurance.

UPPER EXTREMITY FUNCTION

The same medications used for control of lower extremity tone are used when dealing with the arms, with the rehabilitative emphasis on the shoulder. It is extremely important to prevent development of a contracture. Multiple sclerosis may result in contraction of the hands, and the use of bracing becomes important. Once again, keeping the joints mobile is essential. Stretching the digits out at night to prevent flexion contractures is necessary. Using a rubber ball is a bad idea.

Occupational therapists (OTRs) are most generally involved in managing upper extremity dysfunction and the activities of daily living (ADLs). Treatment may involve the use of static splints, mobile arm supports, and other devices that can compensate for upper extremity weakness (10).

No exercises are of real value in tremor management. As noted previously, there are medications that may help. Sometimes devices that mechanically hold the arms can be used for stabilization. Weights may be added to the arms to decrease gross oscillations. Adapted feeding devices may allow for eating independence.

Upper extremity problems are significant, but because the distance from the spinal cord to the legs is longer, lower extremity problems are more common. Nonetheless, the aggressive OTR should focus on devices to aid in writing, dressing, toileting, and other important activities. Technology has resulted in improved wheelchair adaptations along with "high tech" devices to help maximize what can be done with impaired arms and hands.

It is important that the general physician be aware of the services that can be provided by health care professionals that include OTRs, RPTs, RNs, and specialist physicians such as physiatrists. Whether the problem is spasticity management or eating, the interdisciplinary team will be invaluable partners. *The concept that there is nothing to be done could not be farther from the truth.* It is important to realize, however, that time and patience may be needed to obtain maximal effect.

REFERENCES

1. Vital and Health Statistics. Prevalence of Selected Chronic Conditions: United States, 1990–1992, Table 22.
2. Haselkorn JK, Leer SE, Hall JA, Pate DJ. Mobility in multiple sclerosis. In: Burks JS, Johnson KP (eds.). *Multiple sclerosis: Diagnosis, medical management, and rehabilitation.* New York: Demos Medical Publishing, 2000 (In Press).
3. Lance JW. Symposium synopsis. In: Feldman RG, Young RR, Koella WP (eds.). *Spasticity: Disordered motor control.* Chicago: Year Book, 1980:485–495.
4. Young RR. Spastic paresis in multiple sclerosis. In: Burks JS, Johnson KP (eds.). *Multiple sclerosis: Diagnosis, medical management, and rehabilitation.* New York: Demos Medical Publishing, 2000 (In Press).
5. Davis D, Jabbari B. Significant improvement of stiff-person syndrome after paraspinal injection of botulinum toxin A. *Mov Disord* 1993; 8:371–371.
6. Herndon RM, Horak F. Vertigo, imbalance, and incoordination. In: Burks JS, Johnson KP (eds.). *Multiple sclerosis: Diagnosis, medical management, and rehabilitation.* New York: Demos Medical Publishing, 2000 (In Press).

7. Petajan JH. Weakness. In: Burks JS, Johnson KP (eds.). *Multiple sclerosis: Diagnosis, medical management, and rehabilitation.* New York: Demos Medical Publishing, 2000 (In Press).
8. Pal Brar S, Wangaard C. Physical therapy for patients with multiple sclerosis. In: Maloney FP, Burks JS, Ringel SP (eds.). *Interdisciplinary rehabilitation of multiple sclerosis and neuromuscular disorders.* Philadelphia: JB Lippincott, 1985:83–102.
9. Lechtenberg R. *MS fact book.* Philadelphia: FA Davis, 1988.
10. Wolf BG. Occupational therapy for patients with multiple sclerosis. In: Maloney FP, Burks JS, Ringel SP (eds.). *Interdisciplinary rehabilitation of multiple sclerosis and neuromuscular disorders.* Philadelphia: JB Lippincott, 1985:103–128.

CHAPTER 5

Pain

Heidi Maloni, RN, BSN,
and Randall T. Schapiro, MD

Until the 1980s multiple sclerosis (MS) was often considered to be a pain-less disease. It is now known that two thirds of all people with MS experience pain at some time during the course of the disease, that the pain associated with MS may be severe, and that it may have multiple causes. Pain in MS occurs both as a consequence of the disease and as a consequence of the disability that it produces.

Pain in MS is not a poor prognostic sign. Those who have pain as a primary symptom of MS usually do fairly well. As with other subjective symptoms, attitude makes a difference.

In comparing people with MS who experience pain with those who are pain-free, no distinction is found with regard to age of onset, disease duration, disability score, gender, depressive symptoms, or MS subgroups (relapsing-remitting, secondary progressive, primary progressive, and progressive-relapsing). Individuals with a longer history of disease who are of advancing age and experience severe symptoms are more likely to have pain as a symptom.

The following is a review of the types of pain seen in MS and the management of acute, subacute, and chronic pain.

ACUTE PAIN

Acute pain is usually brief and paroxysmal (sharp intermittent spasms of sudden and spontaneous onset). These paroxysms are described as lanci-

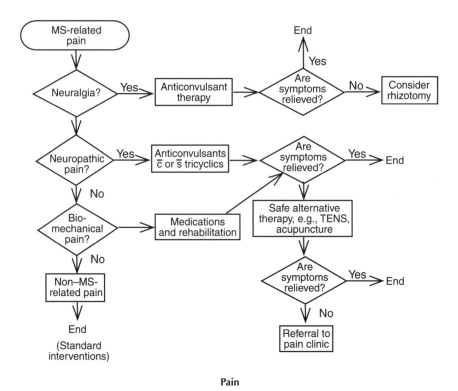

Pain

nating, intense, sharp, shooting, electric shock–like, ticlike, and burning. The types of acute pain experienced in MS include trigeminal neuralgia, episodic facial pain, paroxysmal limb pain, and headache. Any and all of the acute pain syndromes discussed may suggest a worsening of MS symptoms and should be carefully evaluated.

Trigeminal Neuralgia

Neuralgia, the paroxysmal pain that occurs along the distribution of a peripheral nerve, is often lightning-like in quality and extremely severe. The best known neuralgia is trigeminal neuralgia (tic douloureux), which involves the second and third divisions of the trigeminal nerve that innervates the face, cheek, and jaw. In MS, neuralgia occurs as the result of demyelination along the trigeminal nerve pathway within the brainstem. The pain is exacerbated by touching, chewing, smiling, or any facial movement. The pain may be accompanied by numbness of the face. Pain often occurs around or behind the eye and may be confused with the pain of optic or retrobulbar neuritis.

Trigeminal neuralgia affects 2 percent of all people with MS and is 400 times more common in people with MS than in the general population. This type of pain affects men at a greater rate than women. A person experiencing the pain of trigeminal neuralgia may be seen holding his face and jaw rigid and talking with his teeth clamped shut and his head motionless. Periods of remission follow sharp shocklike attacks of 2 to 3 seconds in duration, or occasionally several minutes; in a few rare instances, the patient experiences continuous pain.

Trigeminal neuralgia in MS is often cyclic, and treatment with medication is preferred over invasive surgical procedures. Management strategies include the use of anticonvulsant medications. Carbamazepine (Tegretol®) is the most effective, but phenytoin (Dilantin®), gabapentin (Neurontin®), and valproate (Depakote®) may be helpful. Misoprostol (Cytotec®) may also be helpful. Doses must be adjusted to individual variation, and blood levels may be helpful in determining toxicity. These and other drugs are listed in Table 5-1. Analgesics are ineffective for the treatment of trigeminal neuralgia and will simply exchange one problem for another, as the doses necessary to dull the pain will dull the individual and allow for dependency issues.

Treatment choice is based on response and tolerability. Combining medications is one way to reduce the dose of each drug while minimizing adverse effects. In cases in which pain relief is not obtained by medical interventions, surgical radiofrequency or nerve block procedures that interrupt the pain pathway may become an option. These procedures should be reserved for intractable medical failures.

Episodic Facial Pain

Episodic facial pain is distinguished from trigeminal neuralgia as a burning, dull, aching, or nagging pain. Some clinicians consider it to be a precursor of trigeminal neuralgia. This pain also is resistant to analgesics such as aspirin, acetaminophen, or nonsteroidal antiinflammatory drugs. As with trigeminal neuralgia, carbamazepine is the drug of choice. Monotherapies using amitriptyline, phenytoin, or baclofen are also useful. Gabapentin (Neurontin®) may be helpful.

Tonic Seizures

Tonic seizures are seen in 17 percent of people with MS sometime during the course of the disease. These paroxysmal episodes demonstrate no changes on electroencephalography (EEG) or the loss of consciousness that is typically seen in seizures. Tonic seizures are brief, unilateral muscle

Table 5-1 Pharmacologic Treatment of Acute Pain in Multiple Sclerosis

Agent	Mechanism of action	Dosage	Adverse events	Indications
carbamazepine (Tegretol)	Reduces the flux of sodium ions, blocking membrane sodium channels responsible for action potential	100–200 mg tid pain usually resolved in 4 to 24 hours if effect is expected	nystagmus, rash, fatigue, dizziness, hepatotoxicity, diplopia, ataxia, bone marrow toxicity, drowsiness	drug of choice: trigeminal neuralgia, tonic seizures, painful Lhermitte's paroxysmal limb pain episodic facial pain
baclofen (Lioresal)	Depresses excitatory trigeminal nerve transmission Increases latency of response	30 to 80 mg qd	weakness drowsiness dizziness nausea fatigue seizures	trigeminal neuralgia episodic facial pain
diphenylhydantoin (Dilantin) valproate (Depakote) misoprostol (Cytotec)	Similar to carbamazepine	200 to 400 mg qd	drowsiness dizziness	trigeminal neuralgia episodic facial pain diplopia
gabapentin (Neurontin)	Increases regional accumulation and synthesis of gamma-aminobutyric acid Decreases excitatory neurotransmitter glutamate	slow titration of 300 to 900 mg qd minimum dose, 2400 mg over three weeks to increase tolerability	dizziness, somnolence tremor, diplopia ataxia, fatigue, nystagmus few drug interactions (does not generate blood dyscrasia)	trigeminal neuralgia episodic facial pain painful Lhermitte's paroxysmal limb pain tonic seizures
Tricyclic antidepressant amitriptyline (Elavil) imipramine (Tofranil)	Interrupts the reuptake of neurotransmitters, thus modulating pain pathways descending the spine	10 to 25 mg hs increase to 150 to 200 mg hs	dry mouth drowsiness blurred vision constipation urinary retention	episodic facial pain paroxysmal limb pain headache

twitching, cramping, and spasms, usually of the limbs, preceded and accompanied by intense radiating pain, burning, or tingling. These spasms are provoked by a "trigger" (touch, movement, or hyperventilation) or they may occur in the absence of a trigger. Carbamazepine is extremely effective in suppressing painful tonic seizures.

Paroxysmal Pain

When not associated with tonic seizures, paroxysmal pain is a burning, aching, or itching that lasts several seconds to several minutes. It can affect any part of the body, including the perineum, but it most often involves the extremities. Paroxysmal limb pain of this nature responds best to amitriptyline, clonazepam, diazepam, gabapentin, or applications of heat and cold.

Headache

The association between headache and MS is unclear. Headache is seen in people with MS at greater incidence than in the general population and is usually described as a migraine or tension-contraction headache. Treatment of headache is ordained by the nature of the headache.

SUBACUTE PAIN

Subacute pain in MS results from events that occur because of an acute worsening of symptoms. These include optic neuritis, infection, influenza, decubitus ulcer, urinary retention, and urinary tract infection. Treating the cause usually alleviates the pain.

Optic neuritis or retrobulbar neuritis is accompanied by inflammation of the optic nerve and decreased vision. Optic neuritis is often associated with episodic or constant eye pain, sometimes "icepick-like" in nature. Pain on eye movement is common, as is photophobia.

There may be tenderness in or about the eye. A dull ache sometimes remains after the acute neuritis has resolved. Inflammation and pain may be alleviated by a repeated series of 1000 mg methylprednisolone IV daily for 3 to 6 days.

CHRONIC PAIN

Chronic pain is defined as any pain that persists for longer than 1 month. Chronic pain persists regardless of disease duration or disability. It includes dysesthetic extremity pain, back pain, and painful leg spasms.

Table 5-2 Pharmacologic Treatment of Chronic Pain in Multiple Sclerosis

Agent	Mechanism of action	Dosage	Adverse events	Indications
tricyclic antidepressant amitriptyline (Elavil) imipramine (Tofranil)	Interrupts the reuptake of neurotransmitters, thus modulating pain pathways descending the spine	10 to 25 mg hs increase to 150 to 200 mg hs	dry mouth drowsiness blurred vision constipation urinary retention	dysesthesia
carbamazepine (Tegretol)	(see Table 5-1)			dysesthesia
diphenhydantoin (Dilantin)	(see Table 5-1)			dysesthesia
gabapentin (Neurontin)	(see Table 5-1)			dysesthesia
capsaicin (Axsain, Zostrix)	Topical analgesic active ingredient- hot peppers, Promotes depletion of substance P, which causes a lower threshold of thermal chemical and mechanical nociceptors.	a thin film of 0.075% cream three times/day (over the counter) apply with gloves	initial burning redness mild tingling	dysethesia
non-steroidal antiinflammatories ibuprofen (Motrin, Advil) naproxen (Naprosyn)	Antiinflammatory inhibits prostaglandin synthesis	200 to 800 mg tid 250 to 500 mg bid	headache drowsiness dizziness peripheral edema ringing in ears GI upset nausea	back pain
baclofen (Lioresal)	(see Table 5-1)			

flexor/extensor spasm		
tizanidine (Zanaflex) sedation drowsiness hypotension	Reduces excitability flexor/extensor spasm transmission in cord	2 to 4 mg Slow titration to 20 mg qd
diazepam (Valium) sedation drowsiness memory disturbances drug tolerance/dependability	Activates GABA α-receptors back pain Increases presynaptic flexor/extensor spasm inhibition in cord Reduces spontaneous firing	2 to 5 mg pm or hs

Dysesthetic Extremity Pain

Dysesthetic extremity pain is the most common chronic pain syndrome seen in MS. It occurs predominantly in people who have lower disability scores and is characterized as a "burning" type of pain. This persistent type of pain, which often affects the legs and feet but may also occur on the arms and the trunk, is described as prickling, tingling, tight, dull, and associated with warmth. Extremity pain is attributed to demyelinating lesions in the posterior columns of the spinal cord. This type of pain is of moderate intensity, generally tolerated, and considered "nagging." Dysesthetic extremity pain is often worse at night and after exercise. Pain may be aggravated by temperature elevations or changes in weather. Amitriptyline, imipramine, or desipramine in quite low doses are considered first-line treatment for dysesthetic extremity pain. Capsaicin reduces the burning and tingling of dysesthetic pain by interfering with pain transmission in the periphery. This type of pain is frustrating for both the person with MS and the clinician because treatment options do not always bring long-term pain relief.

Gabapentin (Neurontin®) given in sufficient doses (up to 3000 mg per day) has been particularly helpful. Carbamazepine and phenytoin have been gold standards. The older tricyclic antidepressants (e.g., amitriptyline) are excellent adjuvant pain-modulating medications, especially at night when their sedative side effects can be taken to advantage. Dull aching pain responds best to tricyclics, least to gabapentin. Acupuncture occasionally is of value in some people, but experience has not been as good as was hoped. These modalities may be worth a try in interested individuals, perhaps invoking the placebo effect. Biofeedback and transcutaneous electric nerve stimulation (TENS) have had similar disappointing results. Critical objectives in pain management may be achieved by creatively working with patients in a trial and error approach to achieve comfort, which may involve the use of both traditional and alternative therapies.

Chronic Back Pain

Chronic back pain in patients with MS is most often the result of the mechanical stress put on the muscles, bones, and joints because of disability. Back pain may also occur as a result of osteoporosis or demyelinating lesions in the spinal cord and may be accompanied by pain in the buttocks, hips, and/or legs. Any pain radiating below the knee to the ankle should be investigated to rule out degenerative disc disease or disc herniation—it should not be *assumed* to be caused by MS. However, acute radicular pain may be due to MS itself.

Back pain is often the result of postural abnormalities, a weakened torso, the ache of sitting or standing too long, or the compensatory use of muscles to lift and move weakened limbs. Nonsteroidal antiinflammatory agents such as ibuprofen and naproxen are the pharmacologic agents of choice for back pain. Heat, cold, position change, and firm support when sitting or sleeping may ameliorate pain of structural cause. Aggressive physical therapy becomes critical because issues of gait aids, the use of an ankle-foot orthosis, exercise for maintaining strength and posture, and safety considerations all impact back pain.

Pain that is due to orthopedic and other musculoskeletal problems occurs frequently in MS, often resulting from unusual gait patterns with stress on joints and ligaments. Normalizing the pattern often results in alleviation of the pain. Treatments must be directed toward the problem, not the symptom.

Back and joint pain in MS are often aggravated by impairment of mobility, which makes it difficult to "limp" or sustain postures that serve to protect tender spots in people without MS. With poor leg function, an exceptional burden is placed on the arms, and in some patients only one arm is available for normal activities of daily living. These residual limbs then fall victim to overuse and repetitive injury syndromes affecting joints, tendons, and peripheral nerves.

It is likely that some chronic pain in MS is due to deafferentation producing "anesthesia dolorosa." Nervous system pathways that are deprived of normal stimuli may begin to act on their own, producing distorted sensations and pain.

Some authorities question the use of nonsteroidal antiinflammatory drugs in MS because they have been shown to aggravate experimental allergic encephalopathy, an animal model of MS. These physicians prefer to use acetaminophen or salicylates for pain control.

Spasms

Flexor and extensor cramping or pulling with subsequent pain characterize painful leg spasms. Painful leg spasms are associated with severe disability and hypertonia. Spasms often are stimulated by irritative foci (decubitus ulcer, urinary tract infection, full bladder, constipation) or tactile sensation. Pain occurs because the spasm is contracture-like in character and highly exaggerated. Pharmacologic intervention for painful leg spasms is the same as for spasticity (see Chapter 4). Aggressive medical treatment includes botulinum toxin injections and the use of an intrathecal baclofen pump.

Baclofen is delivered directly into the spinal canal, thereby utilizing the lowest possible dose. This technique minimizes adverse side effects and maximizes the therapeutic effect. Nonpharmacologic intervention includes proper positioning and support of the lower extremities, reducing irritative foci, massage, and physical therapy for stretching and range of motion. Severe spasms retractable to therapy may need to be managed surgically by neurectomy or tenotomy.

ALTERNATIVE THERAPY

Many people with MS who experience pain use alternative methods for pain relief. These include acupuncture, massage, moist heat, dorsal column stimulation, and TENS. These alternatives to pharmacologic agents also stimulate endorphin release, thereby creating analgesis. In extreme cases, a surgical procedure to interrupt pain pathways may be necessary. People with MS who experience pain can exercise some modest control over their pain by optimizing rest, relaxation, stress management, and proper diet. Exercise programs such as Tai Chi, meditation, centering, hypnotherapy, imagery, and biofeedback are techniques that may serve to improve quality of life. It is important to ask what techniques or approaches your patients may be using, so that they may be taken into consideration when planning treatment.

Summary

Pain is a symptom that demands serious attention, as it has such a pervasive impact on role, mood, capacity to work and rest, and interpersonal relationships. Untreated pain causes isolation, anger, and depression. Optimum therapeutic treatment involves a commitment to the goal of controlling pain and improving quality of life.

People with MS are not immune to other causes of pain and it should not be assumed that pain is always due to MS. All too often problems are ascribed to MS that in fact have other causes and require other treatments.

REFERENCES

1. Paty D, Hashimoto S, Evers G. Management of multiple sclerosis and interpretation of clinical trials. In: Paty D, Ebers G (eds.). *Multiple sclerosis.* Philadelphia: FA Davis, 1998:445–447.
2. Compston A. Treatment and management of multiple sclerosis. In: Compston A (ed.). *McAlpine's multiple sclerosis.* London: Churchill Livingstone, 1998:456–457.
3. Clanet M, Azais-Vuillemin C. What is new in the symptomatic management of multiple sclerosis. In: Thompson A, Polman C, Hohlfeld T (eds.). *Multiple sclerosis: Clinical challenges and controversies.* London: Martin Dunitz, 1997:237–238.

CHAPTER **6**

Bladder Dysfunction

Kathleen C. Kobashi, MD,
and Gary E. Leach, MD

Multiple sclerosis (MS) involves focal neural demyelination with relative sparing of axons and resultant impaired nerve conduction. Demyelination commonly affects the posterolateral columns of the spinal cord, with the majority of patients having cervical cord involvement. Forty percent of patients have lumbar cord involvement and 18 percent have sacral cord involvement. The cerebral cortex and midbrain may also be affected. Lesions in any of these areas can affect voiding function.

Fifty percent to 90 percent of all MS patients will experience bladder dysfunction during the course of the disease (1–3), and voiding dysfunction is the presenting symptom in 10 percent of patients (3). Therefore, it is imperative that one consider MS in the differential diagnosis of patients with significant voiding complaints.

BLADDER DYSFUNCTION IN MULTIPLE SCLEROSIS PATIENTS

The incidence of bladder dysfunction in MS patients is shown in Table 6-1. Urinary incontinence related to neurogenic bladder dysfunction is caused by one of three problems: (1) failure to store, (2) failure to empty, or (3) a combination of the two (Table 6-2). It is important to rule out urinary tract infection and other nonneurogenic causes, particularly in multiparous women who may have gynecologic causes for incontinence.

Table 6-1. Incidence of Bladder Function Abnormalities in MS Patients

ABNORMALITY	INCIDENCE
	Range (average)
Detrusor hyperreflexia, sphincter synergia	26%–50% (38%)
Detrusor hyperreflexia, sphincter dyssynergia	24%–46% (29%)
Arreflexia	19%–40% (26%)

Causes of failure to store include detrusor hyperreflexia, the most common urodynamic abnormality found in MS patients. Detrusor hyperreflexia is defined as involuntary bladder contraction in a patient with a known neurologic abnormality such as MS. It involves overactivity of the detrusor muscle, which results in symptoms of urgency and often urge incontinence. The incidence of detrusor hyperreflexia in MS patients with urinary symptoms is 50 percent to 99 percent. Thirty percent to 65 percent of patients with detrusor hyperreflexia have coexistent striated sphincter dyssynergia, which is termed *detrusor-sphincter dyssynergia*. This is a condition in which the striated urethral sphincter closes when the detrusor contracts.

Detrusor-sphincter dyssynergia may result in increased intravesical pressure and an increased risk of kidney damage. Sustained high intravesical pressures may result in urologic complications such as hydronephro-

Table 6-2. Bladder Dysfunction and Presenting Symptoms

BLADDER DYSFUNCTION	SYMPTOMS
Failure of urine storage	
• Detrusor hyperreflexia	Urgency
	Frequency
	± Urge incontinence
Failure of bladder emptying	
• Acontractile bladder	Urinary retention
	Urinary tract infection
	Overflow incontinence
• Detrusor hyperreflexia with poorly sustained contractions	
Or	
• Detrusor-sphincter dyssynergia	Urgency
	Frequency
	± Urge incontinence
	Urinary retention
	Urinary tract infection
	Obstructive symptoms

sis or impairment of renal function. The threat of urologic complications is less likely in the absence of sustained high pressures during voiding or storage and low post-void residuals. Upper urinary tract complications such as hydronephrosis, renal insufficiency, or renal failure have been reported in 15 percent to 20 percent of MS patients with bladder dysfunction (4). Conditions that may predispose patients to urologic complications include detrusor-sphincter dyssynergia, poor bladder compliance as demonstrated by detrusor filling pressure >40 cm H_2O, or an indwelling Foley catheter (4,5).

Failure of bladder emptying includes an acontractile bladder, which occurs in 5 percent to 20 percent of patients (3). Patients with an acontractile bladder may present with a variety of clinical pictures, including incomplete emptying, a total inability to void, recurrent urinary tract infections, urinary urgency, urge incontinence, and overflow incontinence. Detrusor acontractility typically results in a low-pressure urinary retention. However, over time, the detrusor compliance may deteriorate. Intravesical pressures may then be elevated even at low volumes. Low bladder compliance can therefore result in inhibited upper tract emptying, hydronephrosis, renal insufficiency, incontinence, and urinary tract infections (6).

Failure to store, with features of failure to empty, includes (1) detrusor-sphincter dyssynergia and (2) impaired contractility with or without concomitant dyssynergia, a clinical picture similar to the detrusor hyperreflexia with impaired contractility seen in the geriatric patient population (7). Sixty percent of MS patients suffer from a combination of suboptimal urine storage and bladder emptying. Patients in this group tend to have symptoms of urgency with incomplete bladder emptying.

PRESENTATION AND EVALUATION

History

The most common presenting urologic complaints are urgency, frequency, and urge incontinence. Irritative symptoms occur in approximately 65 percent of MS patients with voiding complaints (8). As mentioned previously, bladder dysfunction may be categorized as problems of urine storage and bladder emptying. Twenty-five percent present with urinary retention or obstructive symptoms, including decreased force of stream, hesitancy, intermittency, double voiding, or straining to void. Ten percent describe a combination of both irritative and obstructive symptoms. Patients also often have a history of recurrent urinary tract infections.

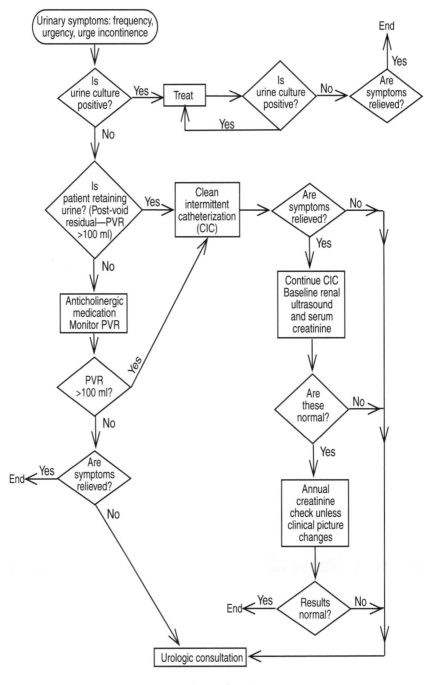

Bladder Dysfunction

Physical Examination

A focused neurologic examination is imperative because MS patients present with variable clinical pictures and tend to have complex, unpredictable, and fluctuating courses. Anal sphincter tone, the ability to contract the anal sphincter, and the bulbocavernosal reflex should be assessed. Bulbocavernosal reflex is checked by applying pressure to the glans penis in men or the clitoris in women and observing for contraction of the anal sphincter and perineal musculature.

Blaivas reported that 98 percent of normal men and 81 percent of normal women have a clinically demonstrable bulbocavernosal reflex (9). In his series of 299 patients, all patients with complete sacral spinal cord lesions also had an absent bulbocavernosal reflex. Patients with incomplete sacral cord injuries or lesions above the sacral level had variable presence of the bulbocavernosal reflex. Ankle and knee deep tendon reflexes should be checked, the presence or absence of clonus and the Babinski sign should be noted, and sensation to light touch and pin prick in the lumbar and sacral dermatomes should be evaluated (Figure 6-1) (10).

Finally, assessment of a patient's coordination, cognitive function, and manual dexterity is important because many MS patients may benefit from clean intermittent catheterization.

Laboratory Studies

Because 19 percent to 21 percent of MS patients have positive urine cultures before institution of medical therapy (11–13) and many have a history of recurrent urinary tract infections, one of the first steps in their evaluation is a urinalysis and a urine culture. Sirls reported that 11 percent of MS patients continued to have recurrent urinary tract infections despite medical management (3). If the urine culture is positive, the infection should be treated with appropriate antibiotics before further evaluation. A baseline serum creatinine should also be obtained. It is sufficient to check renal function annually if all baseline studies are normal.

Radiologic Studies

A baseline renal ultrasound should be obtained in all MS patients with voiding dysfunction. In Sirls's series, fewer than 7 percent of MS patients with voiding dysfunction had hydronephrosis at presentation (3). Patients with hydronephrosis should be referred to a urologist. Sixty-six percent of patients who had hydronephrosis in Sirls's study had an acon-

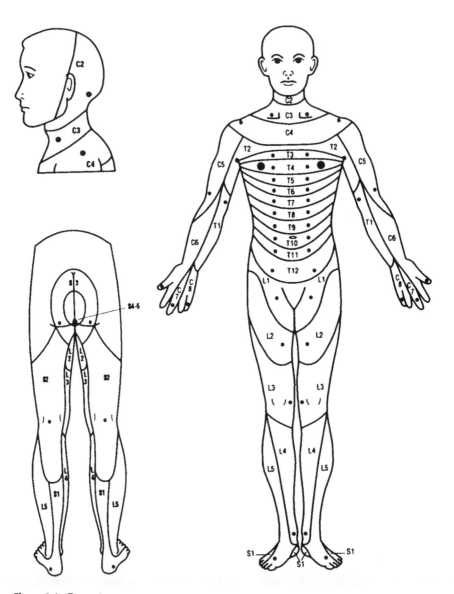

Figure 6-1. Dermatomes

tractile bladder. Hydronephrosis resolved in these three patients follow-ing institution of clean intermittent catheterization. Annual imaging studies are not necessary in patients with a normal baseline renal ultra-sound and creatinine and need only be repeated if their clinical status changes.

Urodynamic Studies

Urodynamic studies define the cause of incontinence by providing valuable information regarding bladder and urethral function. Cystometry is useful in the evaluation of bladder function and may define detrusor hyper-reflexia or acontractility. Noninvasive uroflowmetry involves measuring a patient's urinary flow rate (cc/sec). Uroflowmetry may be helpful in raising a clinical suspicion of obstruction; however, one must be aware that a decrease in flow rate may also be due to detrusor areflexia or impaired contractility. A pressure-flow study is necessary to make this determination and can be performed at the time of urodynamics. Pressure-flow studies involve the measurement of detrusor pressures while the patient is voiding. (See section on potential problems in the diagnosis and treatment of MS patients.)

A primary care physician can perform "eyeball urodynamics" (14) to evaluate for detrusor hyperreflexia or acontractility, which may provide an indication of whether a patient has any detrusor instability and if he or she is adequately emptying the bladder. A urethral catheter is placed after the patient voids, and the post-void residual volume is measured. Next, a catheter-tip syringe with the plunger removed is inserted into the emptying port of the catheter. The bladder is filled with normal saline or sterile water by gravity through the syringe and catheter. The syringe is held perpendicular to the ground, and the column of fluid within the syringe can be observed for any rise, which may represent detrusor hyperreflexia or decreased bladder compliance. Additionally, the bladder capacity can be determined with this study. If a patient has a large capacity with no rise in pressure (level of the fluid column) or no sensation of bladder fullness, this may indicate detrusor areflexia, particularly if the post-void residual is elevated.

Formal multichannel urodynamics adds detailed information regarding a patient's bladder function. Indications for multichannel urodynamics include hydronephrosis, renal insufficiency, urinary retention, recurrent urinary tract infections, and continued incontinence despite initial treatment. The bladder is filled through an 8-French urethral catheter, typically at a rate of 30–60 cc/min. The patient is observed for incontinence, which may be secondary to detrusor instability, hyperreflexia, or poor compliance. Additionally, the patient's bladder capacity, sensation, and degree of emptying are assessed. Electromyography may be performed during the multichannel urodynamic study, although it is not routinely necessary. Blaivas and Barbalias demonstrated a subset of patients with hyperreflexia and detrusor-sphincter dyssynergia who were at a higher risk for complications despite treatment. It is unclear whether this was due to more advanced MS or to the patients' inability to perform regular clean intermittent catheterization secondary to impaired hand function. Conversely, Sirls showed that no patient with detrusor hyperreflexia and detrusor-sphincter dyssynergia had hydronephrosis or an elevation in creatinine with medical management in his series.

TREATMENT OPTIONS

The goals of treatment are to restore continence, relieve urinary symptoms, reverse or stabilize upper urinary tract changes if they are present, and facilitate complete bladder emptying. To accomplish this, a common strategy is to create complete urinary retention and add clean intermittent catheterization for emptying.

The course of MS is unpredictable, often involving exacerbations and remissions. Therefore, treatment should be as flexible and conservative as possible, with the option for modification based on repeat urodynamic studies if it becomes necessary. Additionally, the clinician should be aware that the lower urinary tract symptoms do not necessarily correlate with the pathophysiology of the bladder dysfunction. Therapeutic options for bladder dysfunction in MS patients are divided into nonsurgical and surgical treatment.

Nonsurgical Treatment Options

Clean Intermittent Catheterization

Indwelling Foley catheters should be avoided. The highest incidence of urologic complications in female MS patients with bladder dysfunction occurs in those patients with long-term indwelling Foley catheters (15). These complications include infection, sepsis, vesicoureteral reflux, vesical calculi, severe urethral damage, and hydronephrosis (16).

Clean intermittent catheterization alone may be used when the patient does not empty the bladder completely and intravesical pressures are normal. However, it is usually used in conjunction with anticholinergic medications, which lower the intravesical pressure. One important limiting factor for the use of clean intermittent catheterization is impaired manual dexterity, which may make the procedure difficult or impossible to perform. In this case, several options are available. When feasible, a partner may be taught to catheterize the patient. However, this approach can be difficult.

Various urinary diversion options are also available. These measures require surgery and are therefore less flexible treatment choices than the nonsurgical options. (Please refer to the section on surgery for a detailed discussion.)

Anticholinergic and Antimuscarinic Medications

Anticholinergic medications are useful in the treatment of detrusor hyper-reflexia and may also be used in conjunction with clean intermittent catheterization if any degree of urinary retention is created. In most cases, anticholinergic medications and clean intermittent catheterization are used together; the former can reduce intravesical pressures, whereas the latter can ensure complete bladder emptying. In Sirls's series (3), only eight patients (7 percent) failed medical management and no patient who had aggressive management had upper urinary tract deterioration, including those with detrusor-sphincter dyssynergia. Twenty-five of 59 patients (42 percent) required the addition of a second anticholinergic agent to control persistent irritative symptoms. Alternative agents or intravesical oxybutynin were used in 18 patients who were unrelieved with standard medications (17). Urinary incontinence was reduced in 8 of 9 patients placed on intravesical oxybutynin.

Tolterodine (Detrol®) is a competitive muscarinic antagonist that was released for use in the United States in mid-1998. It is administered at 2 mg twice a day. Because of its higher specificity for bladder muscarinic receptors, its systemic and central side effects are significantly decreased and it is far better tolerated than is Ditropan® (18–20).

Behavioral Therapy

Some patients may benefit from timed voiding, fluid restriction, and dietary modification to avoid stimulants such as caffeine. Behavioral therapy should be used in combination with anticholinergic medications and clean intermittent catheterization and can provide excellent preservation of renal function and quality of life.

Surgical Treatment Options

Patients who fail anticholinergic therapy with or without self-catheterization may require surgery to create a low-pressure storage reservoir to prevent renal damage and/or to provide easier access to the bladder to facilitate clean intermittent catheterization. Surgery may be necessary in 10 percent of MS patients. Surgical options include augmentation cystoplasty and various types of urinary diversion.

Augmentation cystoplasty involves the enlargement of the bladder with a segment of bowel and usually lowers the intravesical pressure by increasing the bladder capacity and compliance. Patients with bladder augmentation need to perform clean intermittent catheterization following surgery in order to empty the bladder and keep it free of mucus, but intravesical pressures are maintained at low enough levels to avoid incontinence and/or upper tract damage.

Augmentation cystoplasty with a continent stoma or complete urinary diversion (see below) is a surgical option in patients who are unable to perform intermittent urethral catheterization secondary to either impaired manual dexterity or difficult access to the urethra. Closure of the bladder neck may be necessary in patients with urinary incontinence secondary to intrinsic sphincter deficiency in addition to detrusor hyperreflexia or low bladder compliance, in whom augmentation cystoplasty alone would not prevent the incontinence. Creation of a catheterizable stoma is preferred over suprapubic tube placement when it is feasible, because suprapubic catheters may potentially result in many of the complications seen in patients with long-term indwelling Foley catheters.

In rare cases such as in patients with a small fibrosed bladder secondary to long-term Foley catheter drainage or recurrent urinary tract infections, severe urethral damage, or pyocystis, the bladder and/or urethra are not available for augmentation. Urinary diversion, which includes conduits and continent diversions using bowel segments, is an excellent option for patients in whom bladder augmentation is not feasible. A catheterizable abdominal stoma may provide the necessary accessibility to the bladder. In cases in which catheterization is an impossibility or when renal function is not adequate to overcome the metabolic abnormalities that may be created by extended exposure of urine to the bowel mucosa, diversion to a conduit may be necessary. Conduits drain continuously into an external collection device that must be emptied periodically. No catheterization is necessary.

CONCLUSION

Patients with MS and bladder dysfunction often present with a broad range of voiding symptoms. Once the diagnosis of MS is confirmed, a patient's urine should be sent for culture. If the culture is positive, the patient should be treated with appropriate antibiotics based on the sensitivity of the organism(s). Once the urine is free of infection, or if the initial urine culture is negative, all MS patients should have a post-void residual (PVR) checked either by in-and-out catheterization or ultrasound of the bladder (bladder scan). Referral to a urologist is indicated if the urinary tract infection cannot be cleared or there is no relief of the initial symptoms despite a clean urine culture.

When the PVR is greater than 100 cc and the patient's manual dexterity is satisfactory, he or she may be taught to perform clean intermittent catheterization and baseline studies are obtained. Referral to a urologist is indicated if either the renal ultrasound or serum creatinine value is abnormal at any time. A urologic referral should be made if urinary tract infections, incontinence, or urgency continue despite clean intermittent catheterization.

In cases in which the PVR is less than 100 cc, empiric anticholinergic medication may be tried, with careful monitoring of the PVRs. If the PVR is ever greater than 100 cc, the above pathway should be followed. When anticholinergic medications provide adequate relief of symptoms, the medications are continued and baseline studies are obtained. However, if the patient continues to have symptoms, he or she should be referred to a urologist.

All MS patients with bladder dysfunction should have a baseline renal ultrasound and serum creatinine. An annual creatinine check is adequate to follow these patients when the baseline renal ultrasound and creatinine are normal. Follow-up renal ultrasound is only necessary if the patient's symptoms or renal function change.

POTENTIAL PROBLEMS IN THE DIAGNOSIS AND TREATMENT OF BLADDER DYSFUNCTION IN MULTIPLE SCLEROSIS PATIENTS

The clinical picture of patients with MS is unpredictable, and the disease course is variable. Voiding symptoms may change over time. Potential misdiagnoses are occasionally encountered that may not be related to MS. Additionally, there are factors that must be considered in the treatment of bladder dysfunction in MS patients that every primary care physician who encounters this patient population should consider.

Bladder Outlet Obstruction Secondary to Benign Prostatic Hyperplasia Versus Impaired Detrusor Contractility

Men with MS often describe voiding symptoms similar to those of benign prostatic hyperplasia. Patients with this condition often complain of obstructive voiding symptoms, such as hesitancy, decreased force of stream, sensation of incomplete bladder emptying, pushing or straining to void, and urinary retention (21) and/or irritative symptoms such as frequency, urgency, nocturia, and urge incontinence. The obstructive symptoms are most commonly due to the bladder outlet obstruction or are occasionally secondary to impaired detrusor contractility. The irritative symptoms are due to detrusor instability in response to the bladder outlet obstruction. Frequency may also be a result of incomplete bladder emptying, which results in a decreased functional capacity of the bladder. In order to differentiate whether a patient's symptoms are due to bladder outlet obstruction or bladder dysfunction, a pressure-flow study is performed (see preceding). "Classic" outlet obstruction is characterized by a poor flow rate concomitant with a strong detrusor contraction and incomplete bladder emptying. Obstructive voiding symptoms in a male MS patient should not be attributed to benign prostatic hyperplasia without evaluating bladder function.

Treatment of Urinary Tract Infections Without a Complete Workup

Urinary tract infections are common in MS patients. They should be treated with appropriate urologic studies such as post-void residual, urodynamics, renal ultrasound, and serum creatinine. Bladder acontractility often results in retention of a variable volume of urine, which may result in recurrent urinary tract infections. Symptoms of irritative voiding may be caused by a urinary tract infection, detrusor hyperreflexia, bladder outlet obstruction, or other lower urinary tract pathology.

Treatment of Urinary Retention with a Long-Term Indwelling Foley Catheter

Long-term indwelling Foley catheters should be avoided in MS patients. Foley catheters are not a benign method of treatment when left in place indefinitely. They can result in severe urethral damage, stones, recurrent infections, urosepsis, hydronephrosis, and in some cases, malignancy (3). Numerous alternative options are available (see "Treatment Options").

Treatment of Detrusor Hyperreflexia with Single Agent Therapy and Misdiagnosis of Overflow Incontinence as Detrusor Hyperreflexia

Finally, patients with detrusor hyperreflexia who do not respond to single agent therapy may be tried on multiple anticholinergic agents or a combination of medications. Treatment with only one anticholinergic is often not adequate to control the patient's symptoms or elevated intravesical pressures. Multiple oral anticholinergic agents [oxybutynin (Ditropan®), propantheline (Pro-Banthine®), tolterodine (Detrol®), imipramine (Tolfranil®)] are available in addition to intravesical oxybutyinin. One must be aware of the use of these medications in combination before concluding that anticholinergic therapy is unsuccessful. Additionally, one should not automatically attribute urinary incontinence to detrusor hyperreflexia. Incontinence can also be a result of overflow in the case of an acontractile bladder either as a primary problem or as an iatrogenic problem secondary to anticholinergic therapy.

SUMMARY

The goal of urologic treatment of MS patients is to restore continence, protect renal function, and improve the patient's quality of life (22). Assessment of the clinical symptoms, physical examination, post-void residual, and basic urodynamics are often adequate to form an effective treatment plan. Electromyography is important in the diagnosis of patients suspected of having MS, but not in the bladder management of patients with an established diagnosis. A baseline upper urinary tract evaluation is important, but annual radiologic follow-up is only necessary if the initial studies are abnormal or in patients with normal baseline studies only if the patient develops renal insufficiency, hydronephrosis, or progressive or new voiding symptoms.

REFERENCES

1. Bakke A, Myhr KM, Gronning M, Nyland H. Bladder, bowel and sexual dysfunction in patients with multiple scleroris—a cohort study. *Scand J Urol Nephrol Suppl* 1996; 179:61–66.
2. Dula E, Leach GE. Role of the urologist in diagnosis of multiple sclerosis. *Urology* 1991; 37:21.
3. Sirls LT, Zimmern PE, Leach GE. Role of limited evaluation and aggressive medical management in multiple sclerosis: A review of 113 patients. *J Urol* 1994; 151:946–950.
4. Blaivas JG, Barbalias GA. Detrusor-external sphincter dyssynergia in men with multiple sclerosis: An ominous urologic condition. *J Urol* 1984; 131:91.
5. McGuire EJ, Savastino JA. Urodynamic findings and long-term outcome management of patients with multiple sclerosis–induced lower urinary tract dysfunction. *J Urol* 1984; 132:713.
6. Staskin DR. Hydroureteronephrosis after spinal cord injury. *Urol Clin North Am* 1991: 18(2):309–325.
7. Resnick NM, Yalla SV, Laurino E. The pathophysiology of urinary incontinence among institutionalized elderly persons. *N Engl J Med* 1989; 320(1):1–7.
8. Goldstein I, Siroky MB, Saz DS, Krane RJ. Neurologic abnormalities in multiple sclerosis. *J Urol* 1982; 128:541.

9. Blaivas JG, Zayed AA, Labib KB. The bulbocavernosus reflex in urology: A prospective study of 299 patients. *J Urol* 1981; 126(2):197–199.
10. Guttierez PA, Young RR, Vulpe M. Spinal cord injury: An overview. *Urol Clin North Am* 1993, 20(3):373–401.
11. Sirls LT, Choe JM. The incontinence history and physical examination. In: O'Donnell P (ed.). *Urinary incontinence.* St. Louis: Mosby, 1997, Ch. 8, p. 54.
12. Mayo ME, Chetner MP. Lower urinary tract dysfunction in multiple sclerosis. *Urology* 1992; 39:67.
13. Gonor SE, Carroll DJ, Metcalfe JB. Vesical dysfunction in multiple sclerosis. *Urology* 1985; 25:429.
14. Ouslander JG, Leach GE, Staskin DR. Simplified tests of lower urinary tract function in the evaluation of geriatric urinary incontinence. *J Am Geriatr Soc* 1989; 37(8):706–714.
15. Holevas RE, Hadley R. Voiding dysfunction with nontraumatic neurologic disease. AUA Update Series, Volume IX, Lesson 38, 1992.
16. Kennelly MJ, Rudy DC. Incontinence caused by neurologic disease. In: O'Donnell P (ed.). *Urinary incontinence.* St. Louis: Mosby, 1997, Ch. 47, p. 338.
17. Weese D, Roskamp D, Leach GE, Zimmern PE. Intravesical oxybutynin chloride: Experience with 42 patients. *Urology* 1993; 41(6):527.
18. Abrams P, Freeman R, Anderstrom C, Mattiasson A. Tolterodine, a new antimuscarinic agent: As effective but better tolerated than oxybutynin in patients with an overactive bladder. *Br J Urol* 1998 81(6):801–810.
19. Gillberg PG, Sudnquist S. Comparison of the in vitro and in vivo profiles of tolterodine with those of subtype-selective muscarinic receptor antagonists. *Eur J Pharm* 1998; 349(2–3):285–292.
20. Hills CJ, Winter SA, Balfour JA. Tolterodine. *Drugs* 1998; 55(6):813–820.
21. Wein AJ. Evaluation of treatment response in benign prostatic hyperplasia. AUA Update Series, Volume X, Lesson 9, 1991.
22. Andrews KL, Husmann DA. Bladder dysfunction and management in multiple sclerosis. *Mayo Clin Proc* 1997; 72(12):1176–1183.

CHAPTER 7

Bowel Management

Nancy J. Holland, EdD, RN

Bowel dysfunction is common in multiple sclerosis (MS) and is reported by approximately 60 percent of those with the disease. The mechanism of defecation is similar to that of micturition, involving afferent fibers entering the S3–5 segments of the spinal cord. Distention of the rectal walls provides the stimulus for defecation, resulting in contraction of the rectal muscles and relaxation of the internal anal sphincter. Abdominal muscle contraction (controlled by the T6–12 spinal cord segments) facilitates evacuation, and voluntary relaxation of the external anal sphincter completes the process. Demyelination along one or more points of the central nervous system (CNS) component of this process leads to difficulties with bowel function. Both constipation and involuntary bowel movements may occur, with constipation being by far the more frequent complaint.

CAUSES AND MANAGEMENT OF CONSTIPATION

A number of factors may cause or exacerbate constipation:

⊃ Demyelination along the CNS pathway responsible for defecation

⊃ Weakened abdominal muscles

⊃ Medications used to treat concomitant problems

⊃ Inadequate fluid intake

⊃ Insufficient dietary bulk

⊃ Decreased mobility

⊃ Pubococcygeal spasticity

Constipation can be reduced by a stepwise process beginning with a search for possible iatrogenic factors (side effects of medications), assessment for the presence of neurogenic bladder dysfunction, then progressing through basic natural measures such as fluid and dietary intake, to mechanical techniques such as digital stimulation and enemas, and finally moving into medical interventions if necessary (see algorithm). Sufficient time (up to 4 weeks) should be allowed for each of the regimens discussed before moving to the next step. This will permit a true evaluation of effectiveness. More extreme surgical procedures are indicated in rare cases and should be addressed by a gastroenterologist.

An overall assessment of past and current bowel function should be done when changes in bowel function are first noted and at least annually in the absence of obvious deviations. This should include a history of bowel patterns, symptoms, and interventions, both successful and unsuccessful. Physical evaluation is also necessary and should include abdominal palpation and rectal exam with assessment of sphincter tone. Assessment needs to further address more MS-specific issues such as medications that affect bowel function and the potential impact of urinary tract dysfunction.

MEASURES TO EVALUATE
AND MANAGE CONSTIPATION

Medication Review

Several categories of medication can precipitate or exacerbate constipation, and a review of medications should be the first step in evaluating constipation. These include:

⊃ Antihypertensives

⊃ Analgesics/narcotics

⊃ Tricyclic antidepressants

⊃ Antacids

⊃ Iron supplements

⊃ Anticholinergics

⊃ Sedatives/tranquilizers

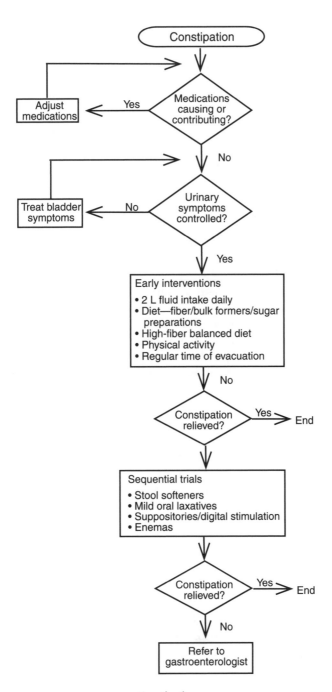

Constipation

⊃ Some antibiotics

⊃ Diuretics

Drugs used to control a hyperactive detrusor muscle (see Chapter 6) are most likely to cause a problem. Medications such as propantheline bromide and imipramine, which often successfully manage bladder storage dysfunction, can contribute to constipation, requiring a careful trial and error approach. Substitution or adjustment of dosage must be done one item at a time, allowing a sufficient interim period to evaluate the impact of each intervention. This effort, as with most interventions to manage constipation, requires patience on the part of both the person with MS and the clinician.

BLADDER MANAGEMENT AND FLUID INTAKE

The next step is to investigate whether urinary symptoms are also present. If both bowel and bladder dysfunction are identified, bladder problems should be addressed first in most cases. Many patients practice fluid restriction, sometimes to an extreme degree, in an attempt to control distressing urinary symptoms such as frequency, urgency, and incontinence. Once urinary dysfunction is no longer a major problem, it will be possible to work with the patient to increase fluid intake in order to prevent desiccated stool, which is difficult to move along the gastrointestinal (GI) tract and to evacuate.

EARLY INTERVENTION AND EDUCATION

Fluid Intake

The generally recommended fluid intake is 2000 ml/day. One way to individualize the volume of optimum fluid intake is to add 500 ml to the guidelines used to estimate needs of the general public (1), or 40 ml/kg of body weight + 500 ml. For those patients without bladder problems, the necessity for sufficient fluid intake can be addressed at the onset.

Diet—Fiber, Bulk Formers, and Concentrated Sugar Preparations

In addition to fluids, prune juice and/or dried fruits are the easiest, and often most effective, dietary measures. Sufficient dietary fiber is also essential, with no less than 15 grams of fiber needed daily. Fiber intake should be increased gradually and from a wide variety of sources. The subcommittee on the 10th edition of the *Recommended Daily Allowances* (1) advises that whenever possible fiber be added to the diet through the consumption of fruits, vegetables, legumes, and whole-grain cereals, rather than by using fiber concentrates. Symptoms of intolerance should be monitored, with a reduction in fiber as needed (2). If a high-fiber diet cannot be achieved, bulk supplements such as Metamucil®, FiberCon®, Perdiem®, or Citrucel® can be used. One or two glasses of clear fluid (e.g., water, apple juice, broth, tea) should be taken with these agents for full benefit. Metamucil is also available as wafers that are acceptable to some patients who dislike the liquid. Patients need to be aware that bloating and gas from a high-fiber diet or supplements may require 2 to 3 weeks to subside.

Bulk laxatives also suppress alternating constipation and diarrhea, which is common in the general population on an American diet. The diarrhea side of this may lead to incontinence, particularly in MS patients with impaired mobility. Use of fiber as a treatment for diarrhea or a preventive measure protecting from diarrhea should be emphasized.

Liquid sugar concentrates are another natural intervention. They act by drawing water into the intestine, thereby softening the stool. Preparations include Sorbitol®, Lactulose®, and Golytely®. Side effects are rare, and these agents are useful for long-term management (3).

Physical Activity and Other Measures

Decreased physical activity due to MS-related limitations also contributes to constipation; peristalsis becomes sluggish, and weakened abdominal muscles restrict the "bearing down" phenomenon that usually promotes evacuation. Recommendations to address these obstacles are fairly straightforward:

⊃ Initiate and maintain a regular program of physical exercise (see Chapter 4). In addition to its effects on constipation, exercise improves fitness and quality of life (4).

⊃ Schedule a regular time for evacuation that takes advantage of the beneficial stimulus of the gastrocolic reflex; 20 to 30 minutes after breakfast is the optimal time. A simple activity to compensate for weakened abdominal muscles is the Valsalva maneuver (bearing down after taking and holding a deep breath). Bending forward to compress abdominal contents can enhance this effort, as can abdominal massage.

⊃ Education about the normal process of fecal elimination, the limitations imposed by MS, and compensatory interventions is essential to promote adherence to whatever plan is developed.

⊃ Integrate the plan into the person's lifestyle and cultural mores.

Oral Agents

A variety of oral agents are available to facilitate the passage of stool through the GI tract. The most frequently used stool softeners are Colace® (dioctyl sodium sulfasuccinate-DSS, 100 mg), Surfak® (40 mg) and generic docusate (240 mg). These are effective for mild constipation. Mild laxatives, such as Milk of Magnesia® or Peri-Colace®, can be effective as a next step. Harsh laxatives such as bisacodyl should be reserved for occasional one-time use and not used as part of an on-going bowel program.

Suppositories

Either a mild glycerin suppository to lubricate the stool or a stronger bisacodyl suppository to chemically stimulate the rectum to evacuate stool is effective when the rectum is full, but expulsion is impaired by inadequate emptying ability. The patient or caregiver must be instructed to insert the suppository against the rectal wall and not into the stool. Patience is also needed; glycerin may need 15 minutes or more to act, and bisacodyl may require 45 minutes. When significant pubococcygeal spasticity is present, the suppository also facilitates sufficient effacement for evacuation. If the lubricant or chemical stimulant properties of these agents are not needed, digital stimulation may suffice.

Enemas

The enema most useful for a regular bowel program is the mini-enema Ther-Evac®, Ther-Evac Plus®, or Colace® microenema, which contains a small amount of solution in a suppository-like delivery system. Fleet® or tap water enemas should be reserved for episodic use, unless atonic bowel is present in severely disabled individuals. Frequent use of tap water enemas can deplete sodium; saline enemas should be used when these are a frequent option.

INVOLUNTARY BOWEL INCONTINENCE: CAUSES AND MANAGEMENT

Involuntary bowel or fecal incontinence can result from several pathologic situations: sphincter dysfunction, constipation with rectal overload and overflow, and/or diminished rectal sensation. Fecal incontinence is often associated with constipation (5). Constipation distends the rectum and interferes with compliance. Therefore, much of the management of involuntary bowel is similar to that for constipation. However, there are factors to consider first when fecal incontinence is reported (see algorithm).

Dietary irritants such as caffeine and alcohol should be considered as contributing factors, and eliminated when present. In addition, medications that reduce spasticity in striated muscle may be contributing to the problem. These primarily include baclofen and tizanidine, both used frequently in MS, and their dose or scheduling may need to be adjusted.

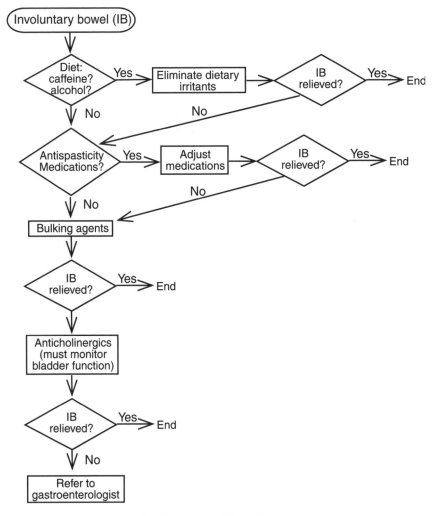

Involuntary Bowel Incontinence

Anticholinergic drugs can be helpful when a hyperactive bowel is the underlying cause of incontinence. Since these drugs also affect bladder function, careful initiation and titration are needed, and post-void residual urine volume should be monitored to avoid precipitating urinary retention.

Diarrhea may lead to bowel incontinence because it is difficult for the sphincter to contain liquid stool. The cause of the diarrhea needs to be identified. Impaction is a common component, with viral and bacterial causes also possible. Since diarrhea can be extremely debilitating, this condition needs to be vigorously addressed for general health considerations as well as continence.

SUMMARY

Most instances of constipation and involuntary bowel in MS can be managed with systematic persistence on the part of both the patient and the clinician. It is important to remember that bowel dysfunction, like other MS symptoms, can change over time, and that referral to a gastroenterologist is appropriate when conservative measures have been unsuccessful.

REFERENCES

1. National Research Council, *Recommended Dietary Allowances,* Subcommittee on the 10th Edition of the RDAs, Food and Nutrition Board, Commission on Life Sciences, National Academy Press, Washington, DC, 1989.
2. Consortium for Spinal Cord Medicine, Paralyzed Veterans of America, *Neurogenic bowel management in adults with spinal cord injury,* Clinical Practice Guideline, March 1998.
3. Harati D, Quinlan J, Stiens S. *Constipation and spinal cord injury: A guide to symptoms and treatment.* Washington, DC: Paralyzed Veterans of America, 1992.
4. Petajan J, Gappmair E, White A, Spencer M, Mino L, Hicks R. Impact of aerobic training on fitness and quality of life in multiple sclerosis, *Ann Neurol* 1996; 39:432–441.
5. Goodwin R, Fowler C. Bladder, bowel and sexual dysfunction: Recent advances. In: Thompson A, Polman C, Hohlfeld R (eds.). *Multiple sclerosis: Clinical challenges and controversies.* London: Martin Dunitz, 1997.

CHAPTER **8**

Vision

Elliot M. Frohman, MD, PhD

Disturbances of the visual system are among the most common manifestations of MS, affecting up to 80 percent of patients at some time in the disease course (1,2). These abnormalities can result in significant disability, culminating in inability to work and compromising the patient's activities of daily living.

Any portion of the visual sensory system can be affected in MS, including the retina, optic nerve, chiasm, postchiasmal pathways, and the visual sensory cortices and their connections. Visual function can also be affected by the development of eye movement abnormalities that result in double vision or the illusion of environmental movement (oscillopsia). All physicians should be able to recognize a number of characteristic disturbances of the visual and ocular motor systems, which may confirm the diagnosis.

OPTIC NEURITIS

Optic neuritis refers to inflammation of the optic nerve. It is one of the most common initial presenting symptoms of the disease, seen in nearly one half of cases (1,3). Optic neuritis may be acute, chronic, or subclinical. Acute optic neuritis is characterized by unilateral vision loss, which may progress over hours to days. Bilateral simultaneous presentation is rare, but sequential involvement of the fellow eye is common. The central visual disturbance may be mild or severe. Some patients are aware of peripheral visual field defects and many notice diminished color perception and difficulty seeing in dim illumination. Most patients have pain in or around the eye, which worsens with eye movement (4,5). Some describe visual phenomena such as flashes of light (photopsias) that may be precipitated by eye movement (6) or, less commonly, by sound (7).

Clinical Assessment

The diagnosis of optic neuritis is a clinical one. Central acuity is usually reduced, although 10 percent of patients have preserved central vision of at least 20/20 (5). It is important to recognize that patients with optic neuritis who retain normal or near normal acuity often have reduced color vision and contrast sensitivity.

Virtually all patients with unilateral optic neuritis have a relative afferent pupillary defect (RAPD) or Marcus Gunn pupil in the affected eye (pupil dilation rather than constriction during illumination of the affected side). An RAPD may be demonstrated objectively by the swinging flashlight test or subjectively by asking the patient to compare brightness of a light source in the affected eye with the unaffected one.

Central visual field loss (central scotoma) is the hallmark of optic neuritis, accounting for more than 90 percent of the visual field defects (8). However, virtually any visual field defect can occur (9).

The optic disc in optic neuritis may appear normal (retrobulbar optic neuritis) or swollen (anterior optic neuritis or papillitis). Retrobulbar involvement occurs in two thirds of patients with acute optic neuritis (5). The normal fundus appearance in acute retrobulbar optic neuritis has inspired the adage "the patient sees nothing and the physician sees nothing." The optic disc becomes pale weeks to months after the initial episode, depending on the location of the lesion along the optic nerve. Hemorrhage at the disc margin is uncommon, occurring in less than 6 percent of patients with optic neuritis (5).

The diagnosis may be confirmed with visual evoked cortical potentials and MRI. The VEP is abnormal in a high percentage of patients with MS and is useful in establishing the presence of optic neuropathy, particularly in those patients with clinically silent lesions. Abnormalities of the VEP indicate dysfunction at any point along the visual pathways from the retina to the striate cortex and are not pathognomonic for demyelinating optic neuropathy. Optic neuritis is the most likely condition to cause prolonged latency, while other conditions tend to cause a greater reduction in VEP amplitude.

Optic nerve lesions are often difficult to see on MRI. T-1 weighted MRI with gadolinium infusion is most helpful in demonstrating late lesions. (10,11).

Natural History

The natural course of acute optic neuritis is variable. Visual acuity typically worsens over the first days to 2 weeks after the onset of symptoms. Decline in color vision, visual field, and contrast sensitivity closely parallel the decline in acuity. Most patients then recover rapidly, achieving most of their improvement by 5 weeks. Some continue to recover for up to a year. The mean visual acuity 12 months after the onset of optic neuritis is 20/15. Fewer than 10 percent have visual acuity less than 20/40 at 1 year (9,12,13).

Despite recovery of vision to 20/15 or to "near normal," most patients are aware of differences in the *quality* of their vision compared with their premorbid vision or to the unaffected fellow eye. In these patients and in asymptomatic patients, persistent deficits in contrast sensitivity, color vision, and depth perception are common.

The risk of developing MS in monosymptomatic optic neuritis is strongly influenced by the number of lesions observed on MRI. Five years after the onset of optic neuritis, clinically definite MS is confirmed in 16 percent of patients with a normal brain MRI and in 51 percent of patients with three or more lesions.

Differential Diagnosis

Numerous infectious or inflammatory disorders other than demyelinating disease may cause optic neuritis (14). Ancillary studies (antinuclear antibody assay, syphilis serologies, chest radiograph, cerebrospinal fluid analysis) are of low yield in patients with typical isolated optic neuritis, and an exhaustive search for causative conditions is rarely indicated.

Acute optic neuritis can usually be distinguished from other causes of optic neuropathy and other ophthalmic conditions on clinical grounds (14,15). History is usually suggestive in patients with compressive optic neuropathy from tumors, anterior ischemic optic neuropathy, sinus disease, and radiation-induced optic neuropathy. Patients presenting with bilateral anterior optic neuritis should be evaluated for papilledema. Leber's hereditary optic neuropathy (LHON), a mitochondrial disorder usually causing bilateral central visual loss, may mimic optic neuritis, especially in young men in the acute stages before the fellow eye is involved. Drusen (hyaline bodies in the optic nerve) can mimic optic disc swelling (pseudopapilledema) and cause visual field loss, but acute visual loss from drusen is rare.

Subclinical Optic Neuropathy

Many patients with MS have asymptomatic optic neuropathy (16,17). About half of all of patients with unilateral optic neuritis and no history of fellow eye involvement demonstrated visual field abnormalities in the asymptomatic eye. Abnormalities in color vision and contrast sensitivity are seen in 15 percent to 20 percent of these patients, consistent with subclinical demyelination (16).

Chronic Optic Neuritis

Some patients with MS complain of visual disturbances yet have never experienced an identifiable episode of acute optic neuritis. Visual acuity is often 20/20, but careful testing of color vision, contrast sensitivity, quantitative threshold perimetry, and VEP often uncovers subtle optic nerve dysfunction in one or both eyes. Most patients complain of either a stable or progressive visual disturbance (14). Optic atrophy, if not present initially, develops slowly over time. There is no current treatment, and it remains to be seen if disease-modifying agents for MS will affect the course of chronic demyelinating optic neuritis.

Neuromyelitis Optica (Devic's Disease)

Bilateral optic neuritis in association with transverse myelitis is known as neuromyelitis optica or Devic's disease. This disorder is thought by many to represent an aggressive variant of MS, although there are distinct clinical and pathologic differences. Like MS, Devic's disease has a predilection for younger adults but has been described in all ages (18–20). Most cases of acute optic neuritis in MS are unilateral, whereas optic neuritis in Devic's disease is almost always bilateral and simultaneous; if the optic neuritis is unilateral, the fellow eye is usually affected within hours to days. Typically, the vision loss is severe. The vision loss precedes the paraparesis in up to 76 percent of patients, but may occur at the same time or after. Primary progressive or relapsing paraparesis ultimately leads to paraplegia or quadriplegia in most patients. Despite the profound vision loss on presentation, most (but not all) patients do recover some vision (7). All patients with Devic's disease have extensive involvement of the spinal cord, characterized by necrotizing cavitary degeneration.

The major threat to life in Devic's disease is respiratory compromise due to lesions extending into the upper cervical spinal cord and lower brainstem. Advances in supportive care have improved the mortality in Devic's disease from as high as 50 percent to approximately 10 percent (19). Complete recovery is possible in some patients despite a period of complete paraplegia. Intensive intravenous (IV) corticosteroids hasten recovery in some patients. For those with a progressive or relapsing clinical course, the choice of immunomodulating therapy is still uncertain. Some patients will clinically stabilize with azathioprine and intermittent pulse steroids.

Chiasmal and Post Chiasmal Involvement
of the Visual System

Demyelinating lesions in the optic chiasm may occur in isolation or may involve the adjacent optic nerve and/or optic tract. With isolated lesions in the chiasm, patients may have more subtle symptoms and findings. Central acuity and color vision may be normal and an afferent defect may be absent. Visual field defects typically demonstrate bitemporal features. Chiasmal enlargement and gadolinium enhancement indicative of active lesions may be demonstrated by MRI (21,22).

Patients with lesions of the chiasm and proximal optic nerve may present with features of acute optic neuritis on the side of the optic nerve lesion, and temporal visual field suppression in the fellow eye (the "junctional scotoma"). Virtually any visual field defect has been attributed to chiasm lesions. Approximately two thirds of patients with optic neuritis and silent cerebral lesions seen on MRI have involvement of the optic radiations (23).

Treatment

Corticosteroids have long been the cornerstone of therapy for optic neuritis despite the conflicting studies of effectiveness. As with other symptoms of MS, the rationale for the use of these agents is based on their immunosuppressive and immunomodulatory effects.

We advise treatment of most patients who present with acute optic neuritis, provided there are no contraindications to the use of corticosteroids. The recommended route of therapy for optic neuritis changed following publication of the findings of a major study by the Optic Neuritis Study Group in 1993. Treatment with a 3-day course of high-dose IV methylprednisolone (followed by a short course of prednisone) was shown to reduce the rate of development of MS over a 2-year period, as compared with an oral prednisone treatment group (24). In most patients 1 gm/day of methylprednisolone may be administered as a single daily IV infusion for 3 to 7 days, followed by a tapering dose of oral prednisone over 2 to 4 weeks (Table 8-1). In young healthy adults, IV methylprednisolone is well tolerated (25) and can often be given in an outpatient setting.

OCULAR INFLAMMATION

Uveitis (inflammation of the iris, ciliary body, or choroid) is reported in approximately 10 percent of MS patients. The symptoms may be mild to

Table 8-1. Steroid Regimens

Agent	Exacerbations	Adjunctive
IV MP	1–2 g IV daily for 3–7 days. Followed by an oral steroid taper, (see below)	1–2 g IV for 1–2 days monthly to every other month

Prednisone	*Taper*
	
	200 mg x 4 days then
	100 mg x 4 days then
	decreasing by 10 mg daily
	  until off
	
	Primary Treatment
	
	400 mg x 4 days then
	200 mg x 4 days then
	100 mg x 2 days then
	decreasing by 10 mg increments
	  daily until off
		Monthly
		
		400 mg x 2–4 days
		
		Every Other Month
		
		400 mg x 2 days then
		200 mg x 2 days then
		100 mg x 2 days...
		can add 10 mg progressive taper

Dexamethasone	*Taper*
	
	12 mg x 4 days then
	8 mg x 4 days then
	4 mg x 4 days
	
	Primary Treatment
	
	16–40 mg x 4 days then
	  (reduce by half)
	8–20 mg x 4 days then
	4–12 mg x 4 days then
	decreasing by 4 mg increments
	  every 4 days
		Monthly
		
		12–24 mg x 2–4 days
		
		Every Other Month
		
		16–24 mg x 2 days then
		8–12 mg x 2 days then
		4–8 mg x 2 days

severe and complications are directly proportional to the extent and severity of the inflammation. Complications of ocular inflammation include glaucoma, cataract, macular edema, retinal detachment, and vitreous hemorrhage (26). Retinal venous sheathing occurs in 10 percent to 20 percent of patients with MS (27,28) and represents active periphlebitis or sclerosis (27).

EYE MOVEMENT ABNORMALITIES

Some form of eye movement abnormality can be observed in up to three quarters of patients with MS. Essentially all known eye movement disorders have been described in patients with MS.

In MS patients, abnormalities in the ocular motor apparatus can produce disorders of rapid gaze shifting (saccades), pursuit eye movements, vestibular ocular reflexes, visual fixation, ocular alignment, and gaze holding. Ocular motor palsies (CN III, IV, VI) have also been described.

INTERNUCLEAR OPHTHALMOPLEGIA

Internuclear ophthalmoplegia (INO) is one of the neuro-ophthalmologic hallmarks of MS and is present in one third of patients (29,30). This eye movement abnormality is produced by a lesion in the medial longitudinal fasciculus (MLF), typically located in the pontine or midbrain tegmentum. The cardinal clinical feature of INO is ocular disconjugacy during horizontal saccades secondary to slowing of adducting eye movements. Despite adduction weakness, convergence is intact in most patients.

Diagnosis

The diagnosis of INO is typically based on clinical examination, in which disconjugate horizontal saccades are seen. Its principal symptoms are diplopia, blurred vision, and oscillopsia (the illusion of environmental movement), although many patients are asymptomatic. Bilateral INO is most commonly associated with demyelinating disease.

Ocular motor palsies involving cranial nerves III, IV, and VI have been described in MS (31,32). Lesions within the pontine tegmentum involving the paramedian pontine reticular formation (PPRF) or abducens (VI) nucleus can produce gaze palsies. Abnormalities in smooth pursuit eye movements are commonly seen in MS (33). Vestibular eye movement abnormalities are also seen and are characterized by nystagmus and skew deviation.

NYSTAGMUS

Nystagmus is a repetitive, to-and-fro movement of the eyes. When pathologic, it reflects abnormalities in the mechanisms that hold images on the retina. Gaze-evoked nystagmus commonly occurs as a side effect of certain medications, especially anticonvulsants, hypnotics, and tranquilizers, and with disease of the vestibulocerebellum or its brainstem connections.

Pendular nystagmus consists of a slow phase that is a sinusoidal oscillation rather than a unidirectional drift. In patients with MS, this form of nystagmus produces the most distressing symptoms, including oscillopsia, poor visual acuity, nausea, disorientation, and instability.

Treatment

The treatment of nystagmus in MS is one of the most difficult challenges for the physician. Many pharmacologic agents have been used, most with only moderate effectiveness. Those that are successful in some patients may be ineffective in others. Such differences may relate to the variability of lesions between patients, involving different anatomic sites and affecting different neurotransmitter systems. Baclofen, clonazepam, gabapentin, and scopolamine provide some benefit in selected patients.

REFERENCES

1. Leibowitz U, Alter M. Optic nerve involvement and diplopia as initial manifestations of multiple sclerosis. *Acta Neurol Scand* 1968; 44:70–80.
2. Kuroiwa Y, Shibasaki H. Clinical studies of multiple sclerosis in Japan. I. A current appraisal of 83 cases. *Neurology* 1973; 23:609–617.
3. Wikström J, Poser S, Ritter G. Optic neuritis as an initial symptom in multiple sclerosis. *Acta Neurol Scand* 1980; 61:178–185.
4. Celesia GG, Kaufman DI, Brigell M, et al. Optic neuritis: A prospective study. *Neurology* 1990; 40:919–923.
5. Optic Neuritis Study Group. The clinical profile of optic neuritis: Experience of the optic neuritis treatment trial. *Arch Ophthalmol* 1991; 109:1673–1678.
6. Davis FA, Bergen D, Schauf C, McDonald WI, Deutsch W. Movement phosphenes in optic neuritis: A new clinical sign. *Neurology* 1976; 26:1100–1104.
7. Lessell S, Cohen MM. Phosphenes induced by sound. *Neurology* 1979; 29:1524–1527.
8. Miller NR. Optic neuritis. In: *Walsh and Hoyt's clinical neuro-ophthalmology*, 4th ed. Baltimore: Williams & Wilkins, 1982:227–248.
9. Keltner JL, Johnson CA, Spurr JO, Beck RW, Optic Neuritis Study Group. Baseline visual field profile of optic neuritis: The experience of the Optic Neuritis Treatment Trial. *Arch Ophthalmol* 1993; 111:231–234.
10. Halliday AM, McDonald WI, Mushin J. Delayed pattern-evoked responses in optic neuritis in relation to visual acuity. *Trans Ophthalmol Soc UK* 1973; 93:315–324.
11. Youl BD, Turano G, Miller DH, et al. The pathophysiology of acute optic neuritis: The association of gadolinium leakage with clinical and electrophysiological deficits. *Brain* 1991; 114:2437–2450.
12. Beck RW, Cleary PA, Optic Neuritis Study Group. Optic Neuritis Treatment Trial: One-year follow-up results. *Arch Ophthalmol* 1993; 111:773–775.
13. Beck RW. The Optic Neuritis Treatment Trial: Implications for clinical practice. *Arch Ophthalmol* 1992; 110:331–332.

14. Beck RW. Optic neuritis. In: Miller NR Newman NJ (eds.). *Walsh and Hoyt's clinical neuro-ophthalmology*, 5th ed. Baltimore: Williams & Wilkins, 1998:599–647.
15. Sedwick LA. Optic neuritis. *Neurol Clin* 1991; 9:97–114.
16. Beck RW, Kupersmith MJ, Cleary PA, Katz B, Optic Neuritis Study Group. Fellow eye abnormalities in acute unilateral optic neuritis: Experience of the Optic Neuritis Treatment Trial. *Ophthalmology* 1993; 100:691–697.
17. Patterson VH, Heron JR. Visual field abnormalities in multiple sclerosis. *J Neurol Neurosurg Psychiatry* 1980; 43:205–208.
18. Jeffery AR, Buncic JR. Pediatric Devic's neuromyelitis optica. *J Pediatr Ophthalmol Strabismus* 1996; 33:223–229.
19. Whitham RH, Brey RL. Neuromyelitis optica: Two new cases and a review of the literature. *J Clin Neuro-ophthalmol* 1985; 5:263–269.
20. Filley CM, Sternberg PE, Norenberg MD. Neuromyelitis optica in the elderly. *Arch Neurol* 1984; 41:670–672.
21. Kerty E, Eide N, Nakstad P, Nyberg-Hansen R. Chiasmal optic neuritis. *Acta Ophthalmol* 1991; 69:135–139.
22. Newman NJ, Lessell S, Winterkorn JMS. Optic chiasmal neuritis. *Neurology* 1991; 41:1203–1212.
23. Beck RW, Cleary PA, Trobe JD, et al. The effect of corticosteroids for acute optic neuritis on the subsequent development of multiple sclerosis. *New Engl J Med* 1993; 329 (24):1764–1769.
24. Hornabrook RSL, Miller DH, Newton MR, et al. Frequent involvement of the optic radiation in patients with acute isolated optic neuritis. *Neurology* 1992; 42:77–79.
25. Chrousos GA, Kattah JC, Beck RW, Cleary PA, Optic Neuritis Study Group. Side effects of glucocorticoid treatment: Experience of the Optic Neuritis Treatment Trial. *JAMA* 1993; 269:2110–2112.
26. Malinowski SM, Pulido JS, Folk JC. Long-term visual outcome and complications associated with pars planitis. *Ophthalmology* 1993; 100:818–825.
27. Arnold AC, Pepose JS, Hepler RS, Foos RY. Retinal periphlebitis and retinitis in multiple sclerosis: I. Pathological characteristics. *Ophthalmology* 1984; 91:255–261.
28. Bamford CR, Ganley JP, Sibley WA, Laguna JF. Uveitis, perivenous sheathing and multiple sclerosis. *Neurology* 1978; 28(2):119–124.
29. Muri RM, Meienberg O. The clinical spectrum of internuclear ophthalmoplegia in multiple sclerosis. *Arch Neurol* 1985; 42:851–855.
30. Meienberg O, Muri R, Rabineau PA. Clinical and oculographic examinations of saccadic eye movements in the diagnosis of multiple sclerosis. *Arch Neurol* 1986; 43:438–443.
31. Ivers RR, Goldstein NP. Multiple sclerosis: A current appraisal of symptoms and signs. *Proc Mayo Clin* 1963; 38:457–466.
32. Rush JA, Younge BR. Paralysis of cranial nerves III, IV, and VI. *Arch Ophthalmol* 1981; 99:76–79.
33. Mastaglia FL, Black JL, Collins DWF. Quantitative studies of saccadic and pursuit eye movements in MS. *Brain* 1979; 102:817–834.

CHAPTER 9

Cognitive Loss

Randolph B. Schiffer, MD

A series of neuropsychological studies during the past 20 years have provided evidence of disease-based cognitive loss in a substantial number of patients with multiple sclerosis (MS). Prevalence rates for such cognitive loss range as high as 50 percent. These cognitive deficits are typically not appreciated or noted by the treating physicians, and sometimes not by the patients themselves. They may be present quite early in the disease course, in the absence of obvious clinical neurologic impairment.

Multiple sclerosis patients with cognitive impairments have difficulty with tasks that involve recent memory, sustained attention, speed of cognitive processing, and conceptual reasoning (1). People with this pattern of cognitive loss typically perform relatively better on tests of language and learning ability. Perhaps because of the white matter distribution of much of the MS neuropathology, these patients perform poorly on tests that access prefrontal, executive cognitive functions, such as those involved in planning, sequencing, and self-regulation. This pattern of dementia has been described as a subcortical or white-matter pattern (Table 9-1). It is more difficult to recognize during routine interviews than is the cortical pattern of dementia. The dementia syndrome associated with MS is also less severe than that typically seen in older patients with Alzheimer's disease.

In general, one should consider that relapse rates or changes in levels of neurologic disability are poor predictors of the degree of cognitive dysfunction. Occasionally patients may present with the clinical syndrome of dementia, but just as often severely disabled patients may show normal cog-

Table 9-1. Cognitive Function Affected by Multiple Sclerosis

⊃ Information processing
⊃ Maintenance of attention
⊃ Recent memory
⊃ Concept formation and problem solving

nition. Patients who enter a secondary progressive disease pattern are especially at risk of demonstrating significant cognitive failure on neuropsychological testing. A few early relapsing-remitting patients do suffer from dementia.

Various magnetic resonance imaging (MRI) indices of cerebral damage are positively correlated with the severity of cognitive loss, including lesion volume scores, third ventricular size, corpus callosum size, and ventricular-brain ratios (2). Recent research has pointed out specific relationships between the pattern of MRI lesions and neuropsychological test performance. For example, greater functional deficits in tests of conceptual reasoning are seen in patients with prominent frontal lobe lesions.

There also is a correlation between degrees of left frontal lobe involvement by MS plaques and poor performance on tests of abstraction, memory, and word finding. Global cognitive deterioration in MS may be greater when the demyelination is greater near the cortex as compared with a close-in periventricular pattern.

IMPLICATIONS FOR MANAGEMENT
AND ADAPTIVE TECHNIQUES

In many situations, our culture is more tolerant of physical disability than of mental impairment. The functional importance of the cognitive deficit syndrome associated with MS can be great in its effect on both human relationships and work performance. More than 60 percent of MS patients are employed when diagnosed, but after 10 to 15 years of disease course this employment figure falls to 20 percent to 30 percent. Cognitive dysfunction is a major driving force in this employment loss and should be addressed by the physician and treatment team early in the disease course.

Unfortunately, we have relatively limited data about the effects of new treatments designed to prevent progression of disease on cognitive dysfunction. The multicenter Copolymer 1 (now glatiramer acetate, or Copaxone®) trial did include measures of cognition as a secondary end point, but no significant difference was found between treatment and control groups. The interferon ß-1b study in relapsing-remitting MS suggested some improvement in visual memory function in the patient group that received the higher interferon dose. Some improvement in cognitive performance was also reported in patients receiving interferon ß-1a.

Agents that may improve conduction through demyelinated regions, such as 4-aminopyridine, have the potential to improve cognitive function, rather than simply prevent cognitive decline, but the data are not definitive at this time. Amantadine and pemoline do not seem to improve attention, concentration, or verbal memory beyond the level of placebo effects, despite their value in MS-associated fatigue. There is also a brief report of short-term verbal memory improvement in MS patients who received intravenous physostigmine and oral lecithin.

Cognitive retraining strategies have recently been adapted from more traditional rehabilitation medicine and applied to MS patients with dementia, but early reports on efficacy are not encouraging (3).

Our best management approach for MS patients with cognitive loss is to provide recognition, diagnosis, and appropriate social or vocational protection (Table 9-2).

Following thorough evaluation of the cognitive deficits present, functional ability may be significantly improved by an individualized plan for restitution of function, compensation with relatively spared cognitive functions, and adaptation using external aids (4). Psychiatrists or neuropsychologists with experience in cognitive therapy are generally best equipped to develop appropriately comprehensive plans. Although preliminary studies suggest that these strategies may be helpful, their overall success and the relative utility of specific interventions in MS patients have not been thoroughly assessed in controlled studies.

FAMILY ROLE

The family may help both the patient and the medical treatment team to identify the need for formal cognitive assessment. Sometimes the person with MS is not fully aware of the functional changes resulting from cogni-

Table 9-2. Therapeutic Approach for Cognitive Loss in MS

⊃ Assess and document cognitive loss
⊃ Define social and vocational effects of cognitive loss
⊃ Administer best available neurologic therapeutics
⊃ Consider cognitive retraining or rehabilitation
⊃ Provide vocational protection and family reorganization when appropriate

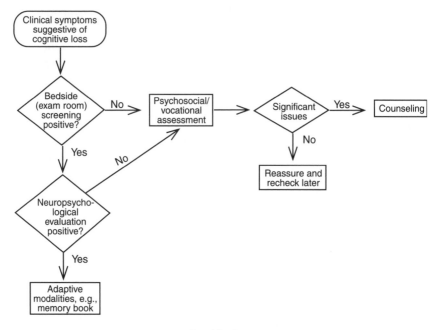

Cognitive Loss

tive loss, and the family can provide assistance and emotional support during the process of assessment.

Some people with MS have a problem accepting cognitive deficits. The notion of disease-based functional loss that is psychological in nature may be more threatening to self-esteem than other neurologic changes. The steady support of family members is key in assisting this process of acceptance and in facing any social or vocational role changes that may be necessary. To fulfill this role, family members must be fully informed concerning the results of the cognitive evaluation, including all available information about the extent and significance of cognitive loss that may be present.

When vocational role adaptation must be addressed, the extended "family" of the workplace may be involved in the assessment process. In our present business environment, such an involvement crosses traditional boundaries of confidentiality and requires the patient's permission. There is the potential for such knowledge to be used against the patient by management in the workplace, as in adverse job actions. However, this risk is generally less for the patient than the risk of separation for cause on grounds of poor performance when management does not understand the reasons for the performance change. In addition, once the cognitive issues have been identified as disease issues, the separation will invoke the protection of disability compensation if the person is unable to perform his or her job.

Adaptive changes in social and family roles must sometimes be faced by people who have cognitive changes as the result of MS. Financial management, family business decisions, and related responsibilities are the easiest to understand as sometimes requiring a transition to other family members. Such transitions are relatively easy to facilitate during office visits when spouses or other primary caregivers are included in the discussion. More difficult social transitions include those relative to leadership roles in families. These may be difficult to identify and alter in the family system. Such leadership role elements might include advice giving and patterns of caregiving. Men may experience greater loss of self-esteem when such roles must be altered. Every family is different, and the treating clinician must individualize the approach.

SCREENING STRATEGIES

The most commonly used bedside/exam room standardized examination in neurologic practice is the Mini-Mental Status Examination (MMSE). Unfortunately, this test has insufficient sensitivity to diagnose cognitive loss in MS (5). Because a complete neuropsychological assessment requires several hours and incurs expenses that are increasingly at risk in managed care systems, the clinician may need to construct a short cognitive assessment using tests known to draw upon the areas of deficit likely to be present.

The cognitive functions that are most useful in the assessment process for suspected impairment associated with MS include:

- ⊃ General fund of information
- ⊃ Sustained attention and concentration
- ⊃ Recent memory
- ⊃ Speed of cognitive processing
- ⊃ Visuospatial perception
- ⊃ Abstraction and conceptual reasoning

Immediate and remote memory and language skills are the least disrupted aspects of cognitive function in MS. Some cognitive tasks that are likely to be sensitive to the deficits of an early MS dementia include a supra-span word-learning task, a digit-symbol association task, and a visuospatial recall task.

A suggested screening approach for MS patients with suspected cognitive deficits might include the MMSE as a global baseline measure, followed by the Rey Auditory Verbal Learning Test and/or the Symbol Digit Modalities Test.

REFERRALS

Referral junctures in the neurologic evaluation and treatment associated with cognitive change in MS patients are shown in the algorithm. These referrals are generally made to psychologists, neuropsychologists, and rehabilitation psychologists. There is always individual variability with regard to decisions about when to refer, based on treating team resources and practice patterns.

Referral During Diagnosis

Neuropsychological consultation to assist in the assessment of cognitive deficits provides a much broader and more standardized evaluation than can be carried out by most neurologic teams. Such consultation is most helpful when there is uncertainty about the extent or pattern of cognitive loss for an MS patient. Occasionally there may be medicolegal issues involved in the cognitive assessment, in which case a neuropsychologist should be involved. When the occupation of the MS patient is a particularly intellectual one, referral for neuropsychological assessment is also helpful to provide a basis for negotiations with the workplace.

Treatment Referral

Rehabilitation psychologists may be of great help in assisting the adaptive process for cognitive loss associated with MS. Cognitive rehabilitation therapies may be useful for some patients, although their scientific value remains unproven. It is difficult to generalize these recommendations too far because each MS patient is unique, as are the psychological resources for any given community.

REFERENCES

1. Rao SM, Leo GJ, Bernardin L, Unverzagt F. Cognitive dysfunction in multiple sclerosis. I. Frequency, patterns, and prediction. *Neurology* 1991; 41:685–691.

2. Comi G, Filippi M, Martinelli V, et al. Brain MRI correlates of cognitive impairment in primary and secondary progressive multiple sclerosis. *J Neurol Sci* 1995; 132:222–227.

3. Jonsson A, Korfitzen EM, Heltberg A, Ravnborg MH, Byskov-Otttosen E. Effects of neuropsychological treatment in patients with multiple sclerosis. *Acta Neurol Scand* 1993; 88:394–400.

4. Prosisegel M, Michael C. Neuropsychology and multiple sclerosis: Diagnostic and rehabilitative approaches. *J Neurol Sci* 1993; 115 (Suppl):S51–S54.

5. Beatty WW, Goodkin DE. Screening for cognitive impairment in multiple sclerosis: An evaluation of the mini mental state exam. *Arch Neurol* 1990; 47:297–301.

CHAPTER **10**

Emotional Issues

Linda Samuel, MSW,
and Pamela Cavallo, MSW, CSW

It is a frightening thing to hear the words "You have multiple sclerosis." Most people receiving this diagnosis will have gone through periods of uncertainty, experiencing symptoms that come and go and vary over time. Symptoms are often vague enough to confuse the diagnosis. Searching for an answer can be frustrating and discouraging. Because of this, receiving the diagnosis of multiple sclerosis (MS) is often a relief as well as a shock. Having a name for something makes it real. Many people have said it helped them to know they were not "crazy" or imagining their symptoms. At the same time, it is a shock to learn that something is seriously wrong, something that will not go away and can have highly disabling consequences. Most of us assume that we will be healthy forever. Losing that illusion is devastating, particularly in early or middle adulthood. Just as no two cases of MS are identical, no two reactions are exactly the same. But there are some common emotional aspects of living with MS that the physician can explore with the patient. These are presented in a question and answer format covering the following eight areas:

1. The most common initial emotional reaction to receiving the diagnosis of MS
2. Common reactions after the initial shock of diagnosis
3. Family member reactions
4. The hardest part of living with MS
5. Depression and MS

6. Suicide and MS
7. Distinguishing individuals who cope well with MS
8. National Multiple Sclerosis Society programs

1. What is the most common initial emotional reaction?

Most of us react with disbelief when we hear bad news. We deny the painful reality and protect ourselves from potentially overwhelming anxiety until we can face the truth. When given the diagnosis of MS, many people remember only the words "You have multiple sclerosis." They remember nothing the physician said about treatment options, symptom management, and support groups in the community. It is ideal if the individual has someone with him or her, who can make notes about the next steps to be taken. Patients and family members should be encouraged to write down any questions they have and to contact the physician for answers and discussion as needed. As in other medical conditions, the doctor has tremendous influence over how a person perceives the diagnosis of MS. Hope is contagious and a positive approach from one's doctor encourages a similar approach by the individual.

Ideally, patients should be immediately referred to their local chapter of the National Multiple Sclerosis Society (NMSS); information can be obtained by calling 1-800-FIGHT MS. Most chapters have educational programs for people who are newly diagnosed with MS and their families. The most accessible and "least threatening" program is "Knowledge Is Power," a series of educational print modules mailed to the individual on a weekly basis. The topics include:

I. What Is Multiple Sclerosis?
II. Dealing with Your Diagnosis
III. Working with Your Doctor
IV. Treatments in MS
V. Disclosing Your Diagnosis
VI. The Impact of MS on the Family

This program by mail allows people to go at their own pace. Another benefit is that they can share the materials with family and friends without the pressure of having to explain MS directly to them.

National Multiple Sclerosis Society chapters also have meetings for people with a new diagnosis of MS, generally over a period of several weeks. These programs offer information and literature on MS, as well as information about other community resources. Those who attend find it helpful and useful to meet others with the same diagnosis. Some people find it useful to take advantage of both the print materials and the in-person meetings. It is important that the person be aware of the available options to learn about MS and to make choices based on his own learning style.

2. What are common reactions after the initial shock of the diagnosis wears off?

Most people experience the diagnosis of MS as a loss. Although there is variability in the process, generally people go through a series of feelings described as the process of grieving. After an initial period of denial, many people feel very angry. Why me? What did I do wrong? How could I have prevented this? Anger may be focused on the limits of modern medicine and why there is no cure. We are accustomed to thinking that disease can be conquered, and frustration is high when it cannot.

After anger subsides, many people go back to denying the disease and pushing themselves even harder. Multiple sclerosis lends itself nicely to that denial, as symptoms frequently remit over time. Some people seek information; others resist any mention of the disease. Denial is a protective emotional maneuver that can be adaptive, allowing a person to continue to function in the face of potentially overwhelming emotions such as fear and anxiety. All people use defenses, and gradually most of them come to terms with the diagnosis and proceed with their lives in a satisfying, emotionally healthy way.

Most people feel reassured to know that grieving is normal and that anger and sadness or a depressive reaction will eventually subside. Giving patients information about the NMSS and programs available through a local chapter is helpful in showing them that they are not alone. Many chapters have volunteers with MS who are available to talk about their experiences in living with the disease. Seeing others who cope well and lead full, happy lives is enormously reassuring to someone who is newly diagnosed.

3. What is MS like for family members?

We say that "MS is a family affair." Although the disease affects one person medically, it reverberates throughout the family. It is like looking through a kaleidoscope—when one piece changes, the entire pattern changes. Family members frequently experience a period of grieving, similar to the process experienced by the person with MS. Fear, sadness, and guilt are common in adjusting as a family. Frustration with the medical field may be a focus for anger. Family members frequently embark on a process of gathering treatment information and encourage the person to see other physicians. Parents of young adults in particular may feel guilty and wonder whether they did something to cause the MS. Families will generally take their cue from the physician, whose encouragement to seek support and information from the local NMSS chapter is an important step in helping families adjust.

4. What are the hardest parts of living with MS?

The unpredictable, uncontrollable, and chronic nature of MS runs counter to the qualities that our culture values. We like to be in control, to know what to expect, and to solve problems quickly. Many people with MS say the greatest challenge is learning to accept its unpredictable nature. Fluctuations in symptoms and fatigue make it hard to plan daily life. The invisible nature of many symptoms—blurred vision, fatigue, incontinence—can lead many people to question their validity. After hearing "but you look so good" far too often, many people begin to doubt the legitimacy of their symptoms and wonder if they are imagining them. With our growing acceptance of the interrelatedness of mind and body, many people with MS may feel pressure from others to somehow "will" themselves well. "If only I were more relaxed, or at peace, or less stressed, hopeful, etc., I'd get well." Such thoughts are both unproductive and unhelpful in dealing with the realities of the disease.

5. Is depression common in MS?

Depression is very common in MS. The uncertainty of the future, coupled with grief over what has been lost, results in most people with MS feeling depressed at least occasionally. Fatigue, a hallmark of depression, is quite common in MS and compounds feelings of sadness and frustration with the disease. Although everyone feels "blue" from time to time, clinical depression is different in important ways. Serious depression involves these common symptoms, experienced for most of the day or nearly every day (1).

- Depressed mood, feelings of hopelessness, and despair
- Markedly diminished interest or pleasure in all or almost all activities
- Decrease or increase in appetite and significant weight loss or gain when not dieting
- Insomnia or hypersomnia
- Feelings of excessive restlessness or being slowed down

⊃ Fatigue or loss of energy

⊃ Feelings of worthlessness or excessive or inappropriate guilt

⊃ Diminished ability to think or concentrate, or indecisiveness

⊃ Recurrent thoughts of death or recurrent suicidal ideation

Clinical depression is present if five or more of these symptoms are present, along with depressed mood or diminished interest, and if the symptoms last for 2 weeks or more. Most people respond well to intervention, typically involving psychotherapy and/or antidepressant medication. Individual and group counseling are often available through the NMSS chapter, in addition to referrals to community resources. The physician has tremendous influence on his or her patients, and the suggestion that he or she get help for depression can be just what is needed to start the process.

There is some debate about the source of depression in MS. Is it an understandable psychological reaction to the diagnosis of an unpredictable illness? Is it part of the grieving process? Or is it directly related to the neuropathology of MS? Researchers believe that all of these occur, singly or in combination.

It is clear that people with MS experience depression for different reasons. In most cases, therapy and/or medication, as well as the passage of time, have been helpful interventions. When depression does not respond to treatment, it seems more likely to be a function of the disease process itself. A few people with MS experience a global change in their personality, cognition, or outlook on life that seems to be disease-related. At that point, help should be directed toward family members and helping them cope with the changes in their loved one.

6. Is suicide a concern in the MS population?

Depression has a continuum of severity. Some feel mildly "blue," some feel the weight of sadness quite fully, and some feel that they cannot go on with their lives. Although people are remarkably resilient, some people with MS lose the desire to live. In these individuals, psychic pain produced by the disease becomes unendurable and isolation reinforces hopelessness that leads to suicide.

The NMSS has supported two national studies (2,3) focused on suicide risk in the MS population. With the goal of identifying both risk and protective factors, the first study produced a profile of those individuals most vulnerable to thoughts of suicide. More likely to be male, they were severely disabled with chronic progressive MS, unemployed, and in significant financial distress. Coping patterns of "completers" of suicide were marked by withdrawal, difficulty expressing feelings and asking for help, and resultant interpersonal isolation. Many of the individuals in the study were virtually unknown by their NMSS chapters but were made known to the chapters by community members.

This profile closely resembles many people with MS who are homebound. Particularly for men, who tend not to ask for help, the physician can have a pivotal role in linking them to resources in the community. Some NMSS chapters have programs especially geared toward people who are homebound, and most chapters can provide referrals to community programs. Participation in this type of program can lessen a person's sense of isolation and therefore increase his sense of hope. Again, encouragement from the physician can be pivotal in the person's agreeing to participate.

The second study of suicide and MS looked closely at protective factors. What are the things in life that keep people with MS going? Does a high level of disability necessarily put a person at high risk for suicide? What can the NMSS do to strengthen protective factors? This study showed no relationship between level of disability and measures of risk for suicide. While suicide completers had shown marked withdrawal and isolation, the second study's sample reported satisfaction, with good levels of support. People with chronic progressive disease tended to have better support in place than those with less severe disability, and they were less isolated. More than 90 percent of the sample had contact with the NMSS in the previous year, and over 80 percent reported that their financial resources were adequate. Thus, social connection and relatedness are strongly endorsed protections. Level of disability does not seem to be the key variable in prediction of suicide risk. Rather, it seems to be the level of connectedness that one feels with others, as well as a positive self-perceived evaluation of one's self, body, future, and so forth.

Almost half of the sample were at least moderately involved in their religion. As we increasingly recognize the importance of spirituality in coping with life's challenges, this finding seems to indicate that a strengthened involvement in one's religion provides significant protection from hopelessness, despair, and suicide ideation.

7. What distinguishes individuals who cope well with MS?

Human beings are remarkably resilient and quite able to adapt and adjust to life. Some characteristics seem universal among the people who cope well with MS. Generally, the more of these factors that are present in one's life, the better a person will do over a lifetime with MS:

➲ Support—People who look to others for support report feeling strengthened and encouraged. The more we reach out for help when we need it, the better.

➲ Connectedness—Feeling connected to others promotes positive well-being. Being connected to understanding others is vital as a protection against isolation.

➲ Sense of humor—Although there is nothing humorous about MS, much of life *is* humorous, and laughter is a healing force that promotes a positive outlook and feelings of hope.

➲ Spirituality—There is growing evidence of the positive benefits of spirituality. Having a spiritual sense about one's life fosters other positive traits: connectedness to others, positive self-perception, optimism about one's future.

➲ Open communication—A willingness to talk openly about MS and the challenges it brings is conducive to positive coping. Reluctance to do so leads to misunderstanding, frustration, and isolation. Families who talk about MS do better at living with MS.

8. What does the NMSS offer for people with MS and their families?

The NMSS has as its mission to end the devastating effects of MS. It offers a wide range of services, from both home offices and chapters across the country, and is available to meet a variety of needs. Educational programs are offered frequently and literature regarding all aspects of the disease is available. As noted previously, groups for people who are newly diagnosed provide information on the disease and available chapter and community resources. Many chapters have medical equipment–loan programs and self-help groups led by trained peer counselors who have MS and are sensitive to the fears of persons newly diagnosed. In addition to these direct services, chapters are aware of existing community resources and the network of support available. People can reach their chapter by calling the toll-free number 1-800-FIGHT MS (800-344-4867).

The physician is instrumental in shaping patients' outlook for the future and willingness to pursue help. Referrals to your NMSS chapter can be made with confidence that the Society is sensitive to fears about the disease and deeply committed to offering a range of programs that will improve the quality of life for people living with MS.

REFERENCES

1. DSM-IV, *Diagnostic and Statistical Manual of Mental Disorders*, ed. 4. Washington, D.C.: American Psychiatric Association, 1994
2. Berman AL, Samuel L. Suicide among people with multiple sclerosis. *J Neuro Rehab* 1993; 7(2):53–61.
3. Berman AL, Samuel L. Suicide risk and multiple sclerosis: A validation study (unpublished manuscript).

CHAPTER 11

Primary Care Needs of Multiple Sclerosis Patients

June Halper, MSN, RN.CS, ANP,
and T. Jock Murray, OC, MD, FRCPC, MACP

When someone has a chronic illness such as multiple sclerosis (MS), everyone involved—including the person with MS, his or her family, and even the treating physicians—tends to act as if his or her only health needs centered around the problems of MS. This often leads to neglect of the health and wellness needs that are important to everyone.

Although MS is usually diagnosed and often managed by a neurologist, the general medical needs of most MS patients are best managed by their primary care physicians. People with MS do not experience *more* diseases than other people, but they do experience the *same* diseases as everyone else. They can suffer from migraine and tension headaches; low back pain; colds, flu and other infections; gastric problems; asthma and other respiratory disorders; visual problems; hypertension; arthritic pains; dizziness; menstrual problems; allergies; stress incontinence; anxiety and depression; and many other common problems.

Also, what wellness needs do we all have? We all need a good self-image; a positive approach to life; laughter, and a joy in living each day; a balanced diet; regular exercise; and general health maintenance through regular Pap smears, breast examination, testicular and prostate examinations, blood pressure checks, and physical examinations. Developing a chronic illness does not lessen the need for these elements of a happy and healthy life.

A recent study of the treatment of 1.3 million patients in Ontario, Canada, all of whom had the same access to medical services, demonstrated inadequate management of other conditions when they were identified as having a chronic disease (1). This is a serious problem in MS, one that is recognized by many patients. When they complain about symptoms that might be due to other disorders, they are brushed aside as being just another manifestation of a disease that can have many diverse symptoms. In addition, issues that relate to good general health and wellness also are neglected in these patients. Every physician treating a patient with MS should pay particular attention to this important issue.

PHYSICAL EXAMINATIONS

We encourage some self-assessment of health status. Women should examine their breasts monthly. If hand dexterity or sensation is a problem, assistance from a partner may be required. Men also need to perform self-examination of the testicles for any changes or lumps, also with assistance from a partner if hand dexterity or sensation makes this difficult.

General health care should include regular general checkups by the primary care physician, with assessments appropriate for the person's age and current symptoms and concerns (2). Assessment of current symptoms and problems, blood pressure assessment, Pap smears, prostate examination, and tests and examinations appropriate for the person's age are indicated.

Although *some* vision problems may be due to MS, we should not assume that *all* visual effects are a result of the disease; all of the common visual problems seen in other people occur in people with MS. Regular checks of vision should be made and those that can be corrected with lenses should be managed normally. MS-related visual problems cannot be corrected by lenses, but the need for reading glasses by the age of 40, and the incidence of glaucoma, uveitis, cataract, and other disorders are the same as for everyone else.

Examples of screening for all people, including MS patients, include:

⊃ Cholesterol once under age 50 and every 5 years over 50

⊃ Fecal blood annually over age 50

⊃ Sigmoidoscopy every 5 to 10 years over age 50

⊃ Clinical breast examination annually over age 40 in women

⊃ Mammography every 1 to 2 years over age 50 in women

⊃ Vision exam annually over age 65

⊃ Hearing exam every 5 years over age 50

HORMONALLY MEDIATED EVENTS

Many women with MS notice changes in their symptoms related to the menstrual cycle such as an increase in fatigue, numbness, or other symptoms just before menses, which improves as the flow begins. If this is a significant problem, controlling the menstrual cycle with a birth control pill may alleviate these symptoms.

It is well recognized that acute MS relapses occur less frequently during pregnancy, and there may even be an amelioration of symptoms. However, there is an increase in the number of attacks in the 6 to 9 months post partum. Many women go through this time without problems, but the risk is greater than at other times. If an attack does occur, it is managed in the same way that any attack is treated.

For most women with MS, pregnancy is a time of relative well-being; during this time families are attentive and supportive. In the first 6 months post partum, the physical demands on the mother are very high, the family attention shifts to the child, and hormonal changes predispose to depression. Help and support in the postpartum months is important for all women, particularly for women with MS

Prenatal and postnatal counseling and support are important to guarantee adequate rest, avoidance of infection, and management of stress. First-time parents need a lot of education and advice, and the experienced mother needs additional support as her other children have their own needs and household responsibilities continue.

Menopause may cause uncomfortable symptoms in many women with MS and can be controlled to a great extent by hormone replacement therapy (HRT). There are other reasons the physician might suggest HRT for a person with MS, as it can reduce postmenopausal complications that include osteoporosis, weight gain, fatigue, vaginal dryness, diminished libido, increased cardiovascular disorders, and decreased exercise tolerance. Because people with MS are prone to osteoporosis as the result of inactivity, HRT may be important to reduce symptoms and possible fractures.

PSEUDORELAPSES

Heat and Humidity

Symptoms of MS are aggravated by heat in approximately 80 percent of patients. When this occurs in a hot room, in a hot bath, or on a hot muggy day, it may mistakenly be identified as an attack, even though the symptoms often disappear as soon as the person moves to a cooler place. Patients often note that they may become so weak after a hot bath that they must lie down for a rest and may even have trouble getting out of the bath. On a hot muggy day the person may be so affected by heat that she feels dizzy, weak, and very ill. Such episodes are not attacks and the patient must be advised about avoiding heat, taking cold drinks and cool showers, and using air conditioning.

Exercise

Exercise is important for MS patients, but some will note worsening symptoms and weakness when their body heat increases. An unusual symptom that occasionally occurs is increased blurring of vision as exercise continues, improving with cooling (Uhthoff's sign). Multiple sclerosis patients do well with exercises in a swimming pool because the water cools the body during exercise, thus increasing exercise tolerance. They should learn how to cope with the heat problem and exercise as much as possible, being reasonable about a balance between the benefits of exercise and the fatigue that it may cause.

Infection

Infections can increase symptoms by increasing body temperature, but they last longer because an infection may go on for many days. Because infections may precede an acute attack, the situation may have to be assessed carefully to see if this is a transient episode related to the temperature and symptoms of the infection or a longer lasting attack that needs treatment with steroids.

Interferon Therapy

Pseudorelapses also may occur when a person first begins interferon therapy as there may be a period during which the side effects, which may be accompanied by some aggravation of spasticity, can feel like an acute attack. In such cases a reduction of the dose, slowly increasing as the person adjusts to the drug (see Chapter 2), usually will manage this situation; if the side effects are intolerable, the person might be switched to glatiramer acetate (Copaxone®).

INFECTIONS

People with MS are not more prone to infection than other people are, except when they develop bladder involvement or when inactivity or being bedridden makes them less resistant to respiratory tract infections.

Viral infections can be a problem because they not only make the person weaker but also may precipitate an attack of MS. Because they do not respond to antibiotics, prevention is the best plan. Vaccinations to prevent influenza are helpful for MS patients, as they, to a significant extent, prevent the major anticipated influenzas for that season. They have been shown to be relatively safe for MS patients.

An interesting coincidence is that amantadine, an antiviral agent that can prevent influenza, may also be helpful in treating the fatigue that is so common in MS patients.

Good general management of infections with fluids, acetaminophen, nonsteroidal antiinflammatory drugs (NSAIDs), and rest can make the person comfortable until the infection has passed.

OTHER DISEASES

Other illnesses in MS patients can be divided into three categories:

1. Those that occur unrelated to MS
2. Those that are complications of MS
3. Those that are complications of treating MS

Common Illnesses Unrelated to Multiple Sclerosis

Illnesses that can occur in anyone else can occur in MS patients, but may be difficult to identify, especially if the symptoms are similar to those produced by the disease.

➲ *Hypothyroidism* can cause slowing down, fatigue, weight gain, slowing of thinking, and even neurologic symptoms.

➲ *Hypertension* is common in our society and this important risk factor must be assessed for in MS patients, like anyone else, and treated if blood pressure remains elevated.

➲ The aches and pains of *arthritis* and *fibromyalgia* are often ascribed to MS. Because nonspecific pain occurs in approximately half of all MS patients, it needs careful assessment to determine how to manage it best.

➲ *Insomnia* is another common problem in the MS population and can make dealing with other symptoms difficult, especially fatigue.

Common Complications of Multiple Sclerosis

➲ *Bladder infection* is a common complication of the neurologic involvement of the bladder and must be recognized and treated (see Chapter 6). Adequate fluids, cranberry juice, and good perineal hygiene are important in preventing infections, and prophylactic antibiotics may be necessary.

➲ *Decubiti,* or pressure sores, can be prevented by good skin care and turning of the patient, with attention to mattresses, pillows, and chair seats.

➲ *Pressure palsies* can occur as the result of pressure on a peripheral nerve, and the sensory loss or weakness that results may mistakenly be blamed on MS.

➲ *Trigeminal neuralgia* occurs in a small number of patients with MS and responds to the usual therapies, including carbamazepine, baclofen, or local neurosurgical procedures on cranial nerve V (see Chapter 5).

➲ *Epilepsy* is not common in MS but does occur in 5 percent of patients; it also responds to the usual treatments for seizures.

Complications of Treatment

Many of the treatments for MS may result in *drug side effects* and *complications.* It is a good principle for physicians to outline the common or expected side effects and possible complications to patients, and for patients to be sure that they understand the drugs they take. Interferons may aggravate some symptoms when initiated, and these drugs as well as glatiramer acetate may cause allergic responses.

➲ Steroids may cause cushingoid features if used for weeks or more, which is not recommended.

➲ An occasional patient who has had repeated courses of steroids may develop *aseptic necrosis of the hip.* The pain and increased difficulty in walking is often attributed to progression of the MS and may result in an inappropriate course of steroids.

➲ *Osteoporosis* is a common problem in older women and is increased in MS because of inactivity and the use of steroids. Recognizing the risks and identifying the problem is important, as this can further disable MS patients and treatment and prevention can be helpful.

Perhaps the easiest discussion is the list of diseases that are associated with MS. One might think that there would be an association with other immunologic diseases because MS has an immunologic aspect. In fact, there is little evidence for such an association, aside from anecdotal reports that might be expected just by the expected incidence of these disorders in the general population. Because there may be 350,000 people with MS in the United States alone, a large number of diseases would be expected to occur due to the natural incidence of these conditions. There is no more cancer, rheumatoid arthritis, or other common illness in people with MS than in any other group of people.

Health Issues for Caregivers

The health of family members who often provide extensive home care services (caregivers) is extremely important but often neglected in the discussion of MS needs and supports. It may be neglected by the MS patient who sees all others as healthy, in comparison; it may be neglected by the physician who concentrates on the more obvious needs of the patient; and, more important, it is often neglected by the caregivers themselves, as they believe their problems and needs are minor compared with those of the person with MS.

Many studies have shown that caregivers neglect their own health. They do not get regular checkups, do not have their blood pressure taken as regularly, and are not being treated for important problems and risk factors when they are present. It is interesting that this is different for women and men in many cases, as women more naturally move into the caregiver role and pay less attention to themselves in view of the new responsibilities, whereas men assume the role in a more organized manner and often organize their own health issues as part of the overall project. Thus, women are more likely than men to neglect their health, their personal lives, and their exercise as part of caregiving.

Caregiving is a natural part of a relationship, and when both members are healthy, the caregiving is balanced and equal. When one becomes ill, the balance shifts and as the disease progresses, the weight of caregiving falls mostly on the shoulders of the "healthy" partner. The number of tasks performed by the caregiver often increases over time, and the caregiver and the health care professionals must recognize that it is in the interest of the patient as well as the caregiver to make sure that the caregiver's health is a priority.

All of the aforementioned recommendations about general health care apply to the caregiver as well. Caregivers should also recognize that the National MS Society has useful information on the nature and role of caregivers and can also advise about respite programs and self-help groups aimed at more successful and healthy caregiving.

CONCLUSION

Multiple sclerosis may not yet be curable, but much can be done to improve the general health and well-being of the person with the disease.

Primary Care Needs

This includes the diagnosis and treatment of non-MS diseases and problems that can occur in anyone, as well as the complications of the disease and the treatments. A positive outlook, a generally healthy state, and an attitude of wellness can improve the quality of life of every person with MS.

REFERENCES

1. Redelmeier DA, Tan SH, Booth GL. The treatment of unrelated disorders in patients with chronic medical disease. *N Engl J Med* 1998; 338: 1516–1520.
2. Hoole AJ, Pickard CG, Ouimette RM, Lohr JA, Greenberg RA. *Patient care guidelines for nurse practitioners*, 4th ed. Philadelphia: JB Lippincott, 1995.

CHAPTER 12

Case Studies

Aaron E. Miller, MD

---

1. A 35-year-old woman, in excellent health, awakens with double vision and a feeling of lightheadedness. Eighteen months earlier she had felt as if she had a "film" over the left eye, which she noticed while applying makeup. Although this persisted for several days before "clearing up," she did not consult a physician. Neurologic examination is now normal except for a left internuclear ophthalmoplegia. When she looks to the right, her left eye fails to adduct fully. Her right eye abducts completely but develops prominent nystagmus, and she complains that images are "jumping." Brain MRI shows six lesions on T2-weighted images, three of which are periventricular in location and greater than 5 mm in diameter. One enhancing lesion is seen after injection of gadolinium.

This woman fulfills the criteria for the diagnosis of clinically definite MS. These criteria require evidence of two or more episodes (attacks) and evidence of two or more noncontiguous lesions involving central nervous system white matter. In this case, the episode of blurred vision 18 months earlier almost surely was an attack of optic neuritis. In the absence of externally visible change in the eye an otherwise healthy young person, monocular visual impairment—which may vary from very mild to severe—almost always represents such an inflammatory demyelinating episode. Although pain on eye movement and photophobia may occur, they often are absent. Spontaneous recovery is the rule, and in mild cases it may occur in only a few days. The current, second attack is manifest by an internuclear ophthalmoplegia. This sign, virtually pathognomonic of MS in a young person, results from a lesion of the median longitudinal fasciculus, extending between the pons and the midbrain. In its complete form, one eye fails to adduct, while the opposite eye abducts fully but develops horizontal nystagmus. This may result in the patient's complaining of jumpy vision (oscillopsia), double vision, or simply blurry vision. Because these attacks have occurred more than 1 month apart, the patient satisfies the requirement for two or more episodes.

The second key requirement for the diagnosis of MS, dissemination in space, is also satisfied here. The first lesion in the optic nerve is clearly distinct from the second, now occurring in the brainstem. Even before the advent of magnetic resonance imaging (MRI), this patient would have met the criteria for the diagnosis of clinically definite MS.

THE ROLE OF MAGNETIC RESONANCE IMAGING IN DIAGNOSIS

What, then, is the role of MRI in the diagnosis of MS? Criteria established by a committee chaired by Charles Poser permit the demonstration of a second anatomically distinct lesion through paraclinical means. Most often this involves neuroimaging, especially cranial MRI, the most sensitive method for detecting MS lesions. Computerized axial tomography is much less often positive and is rarely indicated in patients suspected of having MS.

Suppose, for example, that this patient's earlier episode had consisted of a bout of vertigo rather than optic neuritis. That would have implied a possible brainstem lesion, not anatomically removed from the lesion responsible for the internuclear ophthalmoplegia. In such a circumstance, MRI evidence of lesions in the supratentorial white matter would have fulfilled the requirement for two or more anatomically noncontiguous lesions. Even when there is clinical evidence for two distinct loci of disease, it is now reasonable to obtain a cranial MRI study in a patient being investigated for the possible diagnosis of MS for several reasons. First, with a condition of this importance, one desires as much confidence as possible in the certainty of the diagnosis. Second, the study will serve as a baseline for possible later comparisons, which may be helpful with therapeutic decisions. Finally, it is human nature to desire visual confirmation in a matter of such import.

EVOKED RESPONSE TESTING

Another paraclinical means of demonstrating additional lesions is the use of evoked response testing. This methodology uses computer averaging of many responses to filter out background noise and allow the emergence of distinct waveforms in response to repetitive stimuli in various neurologic pathways. Most useful are visual evoked responses, which may demonstrate subclinical lesions in the optic nerve. Somatosensory evoked responses may indicate lesions of the spinal cord, which otherwise are not evident. On the other hand, brainstem auditory evoked response testing has a very low yield and is seldom indicated. It should be emphasized that the utility of such testing is principally for demonstrating clinically silent lesions. Rarely does it help to perform such a study when the site is clearly clinically involved.

SPINAL FLUID EXAMINATION

Spinal fluid examination may provide additional evidence to support a diagnosis of MS. In this putative autoimmune disorder, several abnormalities may indicate the overproduction of antibody within the central nervous system. Most often helpful is the presence of oligoclonal bands as determined by agarose gel electrophoresis. Other abnormalities include an elevated immunoglobulin G (IgG) index, IgG synthesis rate, or simply increased IgG in the presence of normal total cerebrospinal fluid protein. Although such abnormalities are not specific for MS, they are useful to corroborate the diagnosis in the absence of suspicion of other disorders that are associated with such changes. Although perhaps 80 percent to 90 percent of long-established cases of MS will demonstrate these changes, the incidence is substantially lower in cases of recent onset. Although some MS specialists believe that every patient suspected of the diagnosis should undergo lumbar puncture, most authorities recommend it only in questionable cases.

OTHER TESTS

In a patient such as the one described here, probably no other investigations are warranted. In appropriate cases, however, serologic investigations for such potential masqueraders as Lyme borreliosis, systemic lupus erythematosus, Sjögren's syndrome, or syphilis may be indicated.

---

2. A 31-year-old woman with relapsing-remitting MS has had multiple attacks that included bilateral optic neuritis and unsteady gait. She has been taking interferon beta-1a for 18 months, but had one exacerbation 2 months ago marked by increased ataxia, which improved after a 5-day course of high-dose intravenous methylprednisolone. Neurologic exami-

nation now shows visual acuity of 20/100 OD and 20/70 OS, mild horizontal nystagmus, mild gait ataxia, moderate upper extremity intention
tremor and dysdiadochokinesia, and bilateral Babinski signs. Her
Kurtzke Expanded Disability Status Score (EDSS) score is 4.0. She
expresses a desire to become pregnant.

PREGNANCY AND MULTIPLE SCLEROSIS

Women (or couples) considering pregnancy face several issues. Usually the
patient's most immediate concern is the effect the pregnancy will have on
the disease process itself. A recent large, prospective European study has
confirmed previous data indicating that the risk of an MS exacerbation is
lower than would be otherwise expected during the pregnancy itself, particularly in the third trimester. Conversely, however, the incidence of
attacks is greater than usual in the first 3 months of the postpartum period. Over the long term, childbearing does not seem to convey a negative
influence on disease course. There is no contraindication to either epidur-
al or general anesthesia for the typical pregnant MS patient. Women with
MS may safely breastfeed their babies.

GENETIC RISK OF MULTIPLE SCLEROSIS

Another important concern for many couples considering having children
is the genetic risk of the disease. Although the precise genetic determinants are unknown, first-degree relatives (children or siblings) of MS
patients have a 20- to 50-fold increased risk of developing MS, as compared
with the general population. Nonetheless, this still leaves the offspring of
an MS-affected parent with no more than perhaps a lifetime risk of approximately 2 percent to 3 percent.

THE EFFECT OF MULTIPLE SCLEROSIS ON CHILDREN

Children of parents with MS do sometimes bear psychological burdens
related to the disease. For example, they may wonder if they have caused
the parent's illness or whether they can "catch" it. Furthermore, they may
be fearful that the parent may die of the condition. Sometimes children
will be embarrassed by a parent who has an apparent disability, and, for
example, may not want her or him to come to school. These problems may
be mitigated when parents understand the possible problems. Counseling

or group support for the children or the families may be helpful. Couples should also consider the implications for their family if the affected member becomes disabled. The decision to raise a family is inherently complex and decidedly more so when MS is present. Clear understanding of the issues facilitated by frank discussion with the physician and the nurse may help the couple reach their own best decisions.

LONG-TERM DRUG THERAPY AND PREGNANCY

The availability of the new agents to modify MS disease course—interferon beta-1a, interferon beta-1b, and glatiramer acetate—add new issues concerning pregnancy. First, women should employ effective means of contraception while receiving these medications because none of them is known to be safe for the fetus. Although none has been demonstrated to be teratogenic in experimental animals, the interferons do increase the spontaneous abortion rate in rodents. How long before attempting conception a woman should discontinue these medications is not known, although most authorities recommend no more than a few months. Treatment may be resumed immediately after childbirth if the woman is not breastfeeding.

---

3. A 37-year-old woman was diagnosed with MS after a bout of optic neuritis, which resolved fully, followed 1 year later by an episode of dysarthria, nystagmus, and gait ataxia. She recovered fully and has been symptom-free while taking interferon beta-1b for the past 2 months. She now presented with worsening unsteadiness of gait and dysarthria over several days. On examination, she had prominent horizontal nystagmus, mild dysarthria, right intention tremor, and gait ataxia that requires her to use a cane for balance.

This patient was appropriately placed on interferon beta-1b (Betaseron®) for clinically definite relapsing-remitting MS. Alternative choices, equally reasonable, would have included interferon beta-1a (Avonex®) or glatiramer acetate (Copaxone®). She had done well for 6 months but has now experienced an additional exacerbation. At this point, a decision should be made to stay the course and continue her original immunotherapeutic agent.

At the time of initiation of treatment with one of the immunotherapeutic agents, the physician or nurse should thoroughly educate the patient about expectations of the medicine. This includes not only detailed instructions about how to administer the drug and information about the adverse experiences that may be expected, but also frank information about the results of the clinical trials. Each of these agents has been shown to reduce the frequency of exacerbations by approximately 30 percent. Thus, a patient should entirely expect the possibility—indeed, the probability—of additional relapses despite use of the medication and should not be discouraged if an occasional attack occurs. In the randomized trial of interferon beta-1b for relapsing-remitting MS, in fact, no difference was seen from the placebo group until after several months of treatment. It is therefore not surprising to encounter an exacerbation early after the initiation of treatment.

TREATMENT OF ACUTE ATTACKS

Patients who experience attacks while being treated with one of these injectable immunoprophylactic agents may be treated with corticosteroids in the same manner as patients not receiving one of the drugs. This woman's exacerbation is producing substantial functional impairment, to the point where she requires a cane to walk. Thus, treatment with high-dose intravenous methylprednisolone should be initiated.

---

4. Three years ago, a 47-year-old man had an episode of numbness of both lower extremities that lasted for approximately 1 month. During that time, he experienced some urinary urgency and had three episodes of incontinence. Symptoms fully resolved and no workup was undertaken. He remained well until about 18 months ago when, while on a wilderness trip, he experienced intermittent weakness of his right leg during long hikes. He subsequently noticed insidiously worsening gait, so that he has difficulty walking after a few blocks and must stop. He also experiences persistent urinary urgency with occasional incontinence. Neurologic examination reveals spastic paraparesis, with iliopsoas and hamstrings having 4+/5 strength bilaterally, and diminished vibratory sensation in the feet. Deep tendon reflexes are hyperactive in the legs and bilateral Babinski signs are present. Brain MRI shows multiple lesions characteristic of MS, some of which enhance after gadolinium administration.

This patient fulfills the criteria for the diagnosis of clinically definite MS. He had an initial episode 3 years ago, and for the past 18 months has been steadily deteriorating with progressive spastic paraparesis. Although symptoms and signs all point to spinal cord disease, in this instance the brain MRI provided convincing evidence of additional white matter lesions, anatomically removed from the symptomatic areas. This patient should now be characterized as having secondary progressive MS. He presented initially with a discrete episode, from which he made a complete recovery and remained entirely well for the next year and a half. Now, however, he has been steadily worsening over the subsequent 18 months, without any discrete attacks. The treatment of secondary progressive MS must be considered.

TREATMENT OF SECONDARY PROGRESSIVE MULTIPLE SCLEROSIS

At the present time, no treatment has been approved by the U.S. Food and Drug Administration (FDA) for use in secondary progressive disease. Nonetheless, a number of alternatives are available. Because there is very little, if any, evidence to suggest that secondary progressive MS is biologically distinct from relapsing-remitting MS, it is altogether reasonable to consider the use of any of the drugs—interferon beta-1b, interferon beta-1a, or glatiramer acetate—in a patient such as this one, especially when the disability is still relatively mild.

A recent trial of interferon beta-1b conducted in Europe was terminated ahead of schedule because the drug was found to slow the progression of the disease. A similar trial in the United States and Canada is continuing. Thus, interferon beta-1b may currently be the most logical choice for initial therapy in patients with secondary progressive MS. Based on the evidence from the clinical trials in relapsing-remitting MS of interferon beta-1a and glatiramer acetate that these drugs have a beneficial effect on the progression of the disease (in addition to decreasing attack rate), it is reasonable to believe that these drugs may also be effective in secondary progressive disease.

This hypothesis is currently being tested in a double-blind, randomized, placebo-controlled trial of interferon beta-1a, employing a dose of medication double that which is approved for the treatment of relapsing-remitting disease. A trial of glatiramer acetate for secondary progressive MS performed in the late 1980s was statistically negative. Fewer patients taking the medication did progress, but because the vast majority of patients in both the glatiramer acetate (then known as Copolymer 1) and placebo groups failed to worsen, the trial was markedly underpowered to be able to prove an effect. Before beginning therapy with any of these drugs in a patient with secondary progressive MS, he or she must be informed that the drugs are not approved by the FDA for this purpose and, with the exception of the interferon beta-1b trial cited previously, few data are currently available. Some patients may elect to proceed with other forms of immune suppression such as intravenous gammaglobulin (IVGG) or methotrexate.

INSURANCE

A problem with insurance coverage for these agents may arise when treating secondary progressive MS. Because these drugs are currently FDA-approved only for treatment of relapsing-remitting MS, insurance companies may balk at footing the bill at other stages of the disease. Physicians may obviate this problem at times by being circumspect in their notes about the categorization of the disease process, often an imprecise exercise at best. In other instances, physicians should be prepared to argue forcefully on behalf of their patients when they strongly believe that a particular therapy is warranted.

---

5. One year ago, a 30-year-old woman experienced a sensation "as if she were wearing a girdle." Her primary care physician found nothing and told her "It's your nerves." The symptom subsided after 3 weeks. Approximately 6 months ago, she began to notice brief electricity-like sensations radiating down her spine from the neck as she descended the stairs. These have decreased in frequency but still occur.

She then presented with complaints that objects appear "as if they are jumping" when she looked to the right and numbness on the left side of her face. Neurologic examination showed a left internuclear ophthalmoplegia and diminished pinprick sensation on the left side of the face but otherwise was normal. Brain MRI showed eight discrete lesions on T2-weighted images in the hemispheric white matter with an appearance characteristic of MS. Two enhancing lesions were noted after administration of intravenous gadolinium. The patient elected to begin treatment with interferon beta-1b. One month after starting therapy, she noticed blurred vision in the left eye. Neuro-ophthalmologic examination demonstrated visual acuity of 20/70 with a central scotoma and an afferent pupillary defect.

Over the next year, the patient did well, with no clinical evidence of disease activity. She then developed weakness of the right leg and episodic urinary incontinence. Symptoms improved after a course of intravenous methylprednisolone, but she continued to experience some weakness and could no longer run. Three months later, she developed blurred vision, dysarthria, and unsteady gait, worsening over several days. Examination revealed bidirectional horizontal nystagmus, dysarthria, bilateral intention tremors and dysdiadochokinesia, and spastic ataxic gait, requiring a cane.

She again improved following a course of IV steroids, and when examined 1 month later, she was able to walk independently. However, she continued to have mild spastic paraparesis, mild intention tremor bilaterally, and horizontal nystagmus. Two months later, she awakened to find herself unable to walk. She noticed weakness of her right hand for the first time. In addition to her prior signs, her examination now revealed 4/5 strength in the distal right upper extremity, 3/5 right iliopsoas and hamstrings, and 4/5 left iliopsoas and hamstrings. Vibratory sense was markedly impaired in the lower extremities. She noted urinary incontinence for the first time.

This woman with unequivocal relapsing-remitting MS chose to begin treatment with interferon beta-1b approximately 18 months ago. Although she had an attack very shortly after beginning treatment (not an unusual occurrence with interferon beta-1b), she did very well over the next year, experiencing no additional relapses. She has now experienced three additional significant attacks over the subsequent 5 months. This temporal profile of events suggests that she may be producing neutralizing antibodies that have nullified the benefits of the drug.

NEUTRALIZING ANTIBODIES

Our current understanding of the development of neutralizing antibodies to the interferons and their association with a loss of drug efficacy remains confused. Approximately 35 percent of patients taking interferon beta-1b— and a lesser percentage of those using interferon beta-1a—produce neutralizing antibodies, at least in low titer (1:20) and on at least one occasion. This phenomenon tends to occur approximately 12 to 18 months after the initiation of therapy. In some patients—but it is unclear how many—therapeutic benefit seems to be lost. The situation is confused by the facts that some patients make antibodies and then stop; some patients make antibodies but nonetheless continue to do well clinically; and still others appear to derive little benefit from treatment despite a lack of antibodies.

What, then, should be done for this patient? First, despite a recent course of corticosteroids, it seems reasonable to administer another course of intravenous methylprednisolone, because this clearly is a new and functionally disabling attack. She is obviously doing poorly on her current immunoprophylactic regimen, so a change should be made. Although some authorities may seek the security of a determination of neutralizing antibodies, I would argue that interferon beta-1b should be discontinued and an alternative treatment regimen sought irrespective of the antibody status. Although currently Berlex Laboratories may provide free determination of antibody status, thus making the testing reasonable, there is much less justification for the expenditure of the substantial sum required for commercial testing.

TREATMENT WHEN INTERFERONS FAIL

Glatiramer acetate is a logical first alternative treatment for patients who have failed therapy with an interferon beta preparation. This is especially true for a patient such as this one, whose disease profile remains relapsing-remitting. Although available data suggest that this drug may be most effective for mildly affected patients, evidence does not demonstrate a lack of benefit in patients with moderately severe disease. Indeed, it is likely that any therapeutic agent is more effective at earlier, milder stages of MS.

Consideration may also be given to treatment with intravenous immunoglobulin, which has now been shown to be effective in several, albeit small or flawed, studies. The mechanism of action of this treatment, which has also proved useful in several other autoimmune neurologic disorders, is not known. It usually is administered with an induction total dose of 2 g/kg, generally divided over 5 days. This is followed by monthly or bimonthly administration of doses varying from 0.15 to 0.4 g/kg. Administration of this treatment has been hampered recently by limited availability of the immunoglobulin preparations. Insurance companies may be reluctant to pay for this very expensive treatment, which is not FDA-approved. Other immunosuppressive agents such as methotrexate, azathioprine, or cyclophosphamide have also been employed, but their efficacy is debatable.

---

6. A 38-year-old man with secondary progressive MS has been participating in a randomized, double-blind, placebo-controlled clinical trial of an interferon for 18 months. During that time, his gait has deteriorated so that he has become more consistently dependent on his walker and can ambulate for shorter distances. His legs have become increasingly stiff despite his use of baclofen 20 mg qid. At night he often has difficulty falling asleep because his legs "jump up." His wife complains that he has no interest in anything but watching television. The patient reports that he lacks the energy to do anything else. He has been experiencing urinary urgency, with incontinence two or three times per week, and constipation.

Although his wife states that the patient has no interest in sex, the patient notes that he was having difficulty obtaining an erection. The patient has lost approximately 20 pounds since entering the trial, although he denies that his appetite is poor. He expresses a wish to be placed in a skilled nursing facility because "it would be better for the whole family, since I'm no use to them."

This unfortunate patient epitomizes many of the problems experienced by individuals with more advanced MS. Despite participation in a randomized clinical trial, the patient has continued to deteriorate neurologically. Of course, it is possible that he has been receiving placebo. Alternatively, he may be taking interferon without deriving significant benefit from it. Modern, ethically designed trials generally safeguard patients' well-being by providing guidelines by which a patient may be designated as a treatment failure and offered alternative therapy, without jeopardizing the statistical analysis of the study.

MANAGEMENT OF SPASTICITY

One problem that negatively influences this patient's quality of life is his spasticity. Nocturnal spasms are interfering with sleep and may secondarily be contributing to his fatigue and depression. A more aggressive approach to treating this problem should be undertaken. His baclofen dose should be gradually increased as tolerated. The physician must be aware that higher doses of baclofen may be associated with leg weakness, which may worsen gait. Also, this medication may worsen depression or, at times, produce cognitive symptoms. An alternative medication, which may be added to baclofen or substituted for it, is tizanidine. This drug tends to cause less weakness than baclofen, but substantially more drowsiness. Thus, it may be an ideal medication to add to the regimen at bedtime, especially in someone who has nocturnal leg spasms. Although it is most often reserved for nonambulatory patients, intrathecal baclofen has at times produced improved gait in ambulatory patients, while avoiding the adverse experiences of large oral doses.

DEPRESSION

Clear symptoms of depression are present in this patient. He exhibits a lack of energy, apathy including loss of sexual interest, weight loss, and a sense of worthlessness. Depression is extremely common in MS, affecting more than 50 percent of patients at some point in their course. It may be precipitated or aggravated by interferon beta therapy. Fortunately, depression in MS generally responds well to treatment, and a combination of antidepressant medication and psychotherapy usually is more effective than either modality alone. Although physicians currently tend to prefer the selective serotonin reuptake inhibitors because they have fewer undesirable adverse experiences, in some circumstances some of the side effects of the tricyclic antidepressants, such as the anticholinergic properties, may actually offer advantages.

FATIGUE

Among this patient's complaints was a lack of energy. The physician should attempt to clarify whether this is a psychological symptom, such as apathy, or a manifestation of fatigue. The latter is an extremely common feature of MS and often one of the most disabling. Fatigue may be a result of several factors (see Chapter 3). First, MS patients are not immune to the usual fatigue that can affect any individual. Second, an MS patient, already physically challenged, may more easily "overdo it" and develop fatigue with efforts that would not have been expected to exhaust a neurological- ly normal individual. A third cause of fatigue is depression itself. Finally, a rather unique form of fatigue occurs in MS. Patients develop a sense of overwhelming enervation, which leaves them unable to carry out their normal work or activities of daily living. This tiredness, not drowsiness, is seemingly unrelated to energy expenditure or psychological factors. It is important for the physician to try to dissect the patient's symptoms in order to best determine the nature of the fatigue. The characteristic fatigue of MS often responds to treatment with amantadine. Alternatively, pemoline may help some patients, although randomized clinical trials have not substantiated a benefit beyond placebo. A recent study has demonstrated that aerobic training may improve the quality of life, includ- ing fatigue, in patients with MS.

BLADDER DYSFUNCTION

Disturbances of micturition are another frequent, disabling feature of MS (see Chapter 6). Problems with urination may be classified as failure to store, failure to empty, or a combination of both. Patient history often is unreliable in identifying the pathophysiologic situation, so additional information must be obtained. It frequently is sufficient to ascertain a post- void residual urine volume after the patient has been adequately hydrated. This may be determined ultrasonographically or by simple straight catheterization.

 If the patient complains of urinary frequency and has very little post- void residual, the condition is classified as failure to store and may be man- aged with a variety of anticholinergic medications, such as oxybutynin, propantheline, or tolterodine. Alternatively, if the patient has a large resid- ual urine volume and complains of difficulty voiding, the situation is char- acterized as failure to empty. Although this may occasionally respond to cholinergic agents such as urecholine, it usually requires mechanical emp- tying, which may be safely accomplished through intermittent catheteriza- tion. This technique, performed in an aseptic, but not sterile, manner may be successfully taught to most patients who have intact upper extremity function and adequate vision.

Many patients with MS have complaints of frequency and urgency, sometimes with incontinence, and yet have a significant post-void residual. This generally results from a situation referred to as detrusor-sphincter dyssynergia. In this condition, when the urinary bladder (detrusor) contracts, the external urethral sphincter inappropriately contracts rather than relaxing to allow the normal passage of urine. Initial treatment of this syndrome usually consists of teaching the patient to perform intermittent self-catheterization, in order to provide effective emptying of the bladder, and then prescribing anticholinergic medications to combat the detrusor contractions that result in the symptoms of frequency and urgency. It is critical to provide for adequate bladder emptying in order to avoid complications of urinary tract infection and possibly hydronephrosis and even renal failure.

SEXUAL DYSFUNCTION

Sexual dysfunction commonly accompanies urinary symptoms, especially in men. This patient's loss of sexual interest has been discussed and probably represents a manifestation of depression. However, he also experiences erectile dysfunction, the most frequent sexual symptom in men with MS. Fortunately, the recently available oral medication, sildenafil (Viagra®), often is highly effective and may greatly improve the patient's quality of life. Before the introduction of sildenafil, some patients derived benefit from the intracorporeal penile injection of medications such as prostaglandin or papaverine.

Clearly, optimal treatment to stem the advance of MS has not yet been achieved. The recently available injectable immunoprophylactic drugs are a positive beginning, but many patients continue to deteriorate. Nonetheless, a concerned, dedicated, attentive physician, often acting together with a well-informed compassionate nurse, may help the patient achieve a much more satisfying life by addressing specific symptoms of the disease.

REFERENCES

Achiron A, Gabbay U, Gilad R, et al. Intravenous immunoglobulin treatment in multiple sclerosis. Effect on relapses. *Neurology* 1998; 50:398–402.

Barnes MP, Bateman DE, Cleland PG, et al. Intravenous methylprednisolone for multiple sclerosis in relapse. *J Neurol Neurosurg Psychiatry* 1985; 48:157–159.

Blaivas JG, Kaplan SA. Urologic dysfunction in patients with multiple sclerosis. *Semin Neurol* 1988; 8:159–165.

Bornstein MB, Miller A, Slagle S, et al. A placebo-controlled, double-blind, randomized, two-center, pilot trial of Cop 1 in chronic progressive multiple sclerosis. *Neurology* 1991; 41:533–539.

Coffey RS, Cahill D, Steers W, et al. Intrathecal baclofen for intractable spasticity of spinal origin: Results of a long-term multicenter study. *J Neurosurg* 1993; 78:226–232.

Confavreux C, Hutchinson M, Hours MM, et al. Rate of pregnancy-related relapse in multiple sclerosis. *N Engl J Med* 1998; 339:285–291.

Durelli L, Cocito D, Ricio A, et al. High dose intravenous methylprednisolone in the treatment of multiple sclerosis: Clinical-immunologic correlations. *Neurology* 1986; 36:238–243.

Fazekas F, Deisenhammer F, Strasser-Fuchs S, et al. Randomised placebo-controlled trial of monthly intravenous immunoglobulin therapy in relapsing-remitting multiple sclerosis. *Lancet* 1997; 349:589–593.

Freal JE, Kraft GH, Coryell SK. Symptomatic fatigue in multiple sclerosis. *Arch Phys Med Rehabil* 1984; 65:135–138.

The IFNB Multiple Sclerosis Study Group. Interferon beta-1b is effective in relapsing-remitting multiple sclerosis. Clinical results of a multicenter, randomized, double-blind, placebo-controlled trial. *Neurology* 1993; 43:655–661.

The IFNB Multiple Sclerosis Study Group and the University of British Columbia MS/MRI Analysis Group. Interferon beta-1b in the treatment of multiple sclerosis: Final outcome of the randomized controlled trial. *Neurology* 1995; 45:1277–1285.

The IFNB Multiple Sclerosis Study Group and the University of British Columbia MS/MRI Analysis Group. Neutralizing antibodies during treatment of multiple sclerosis with interferon beta-1b: Experience during the first three years. *Neurology* 1996; 47:889–894.

Jacobs L, Cookfair D, Rudick R, et al. Results of a phase III trial of intramuscular recombinant beta interferon as treatment for multiple sclerosis. *Ann Neurol* 1994; 36:259.

Johnson KP, Brooks BR, Cohen JA, et al. Copolymer 1 reduces relapse rate and improves disability in relapsing-remitting multiple sclerosis: Results of a phase III multicenter, double-blind, placebo-controlled trial. *Neurology* 1995; 45:1268–1276.

Johnson KP, Brooks BR, Cohen JA, et al. Extended use of glatiramer acetate (Copaxone) is well tolerated and maintains its clinical effect on multiple sclerosis relapse rate and degree of disability. *Neurology* 1998; 50:701–708.

Kirkland LR. Baclofen dosage: A suggestion. *Arch Phys Med Rehabil* 1987; 65:214.

Krupp LB, Coyle PK, Doscher C, et al. Fatigue therapy in multiple sclerosis: Results of a double-blind, randomized, parallel trial of amantadine, pemoline, and placebo. *Neurology* 1995; 45: 1956–1961.

Lefvert AK, Link H. IgG production within the central nervous system: A critical review of proposed formulae. *Ann Neurol* 1985; 17:13–20.

Lublin FD, Reingold SC. Defining the clinical course of multiple sclerosis: Results of an international survey. *Neurology* 1996; 46:907–911.

Miller AE. Clinical features. In: Cook SD (ed.). *Handbook of multiple sclerosis,* 2nd ed. New York: Marcel Dekker, 1996.

Milligan NM, Newcombe R, Compston DAS. A double-blind controlled trial of high dose methylprednisolone in patients with multiple sclerosis: 1. Clinical effects. *J Neurol Neurosurg Psychiatry* 1987; 50:511–516.

Multiple Sclerosis Council for Clinical Practice Guidelines. Urinary dysfunction and multiple sclerosis. Paralyzed Veterans of America, Washington, D.C., 1998.

Multiple Sclerosis Council for Clinical Practice Guidelines. Fatigue and multiple sclerosis. Paralyzed Veterans of America, Washington, D.C., 1998.

Murray TJ. Amantadine therapy for fatigue in multiple sclerosis. *Canad J Neurol Sci* 1985; 12:251–254.

Penn RD, Savoy SM, Corcos D, et al. Intrathecal baclofen for severe spinal spasticity. *N Engl J Med* 1989; 320:1517–1521.

Petajan JH, Gappmaier E, White AT, et al. Impact of aerobic training on fitness and quality of life in multiple sclerosis. *Ann Neurol* 1996; 39:432–441.

Poser CM, Paty DW, Scheinberg L, et al. New diagnostic criteria for multiple sclerosis: Guidelines for research protocols. *Ann Neurol* 1983; 13:227–231.

Sadovnick AD, Baird PA, Ward RH. Multiple sclerosis: Updated risks for relatives. *Am J Med Genet* 1988; 29:533–541.

Sadovnik AD, Bulman D, Ebers GC. Parent-child concordance in multiple sclerosis. *Ann Neurol* 1991; 29:252–255.

Schapiro RT. *Symptom management in multiple sclerosis,* 3rd ed. New York: Demos Medical Publishing, 1998.

Schiffer RB. The spectrum of depression in multiple sclerosis. An approach for clinical management. *Arch Neurol* 1987; 44:596–599.

Sorensen PS, Wanscher B, Jensen CV, et al. Intravenous immunoglobulin G reduces MRI activity in relapsing multiple sclerosis. *Neurology* 1998; 50:1273–1281.

Thompson AJ, Kennard C, Swash M, et al. Relative efficacy of intravenous methylprednisolone and ACTH in the treatment of acute relapse in MS. *Neurology* 1989; 39:969–971.

Tourtellotte WW, Potvin AR, Fleming JO, et al. Multiple sclerosis: Measurement and validation of central nervous system IgG synthesis rate. *Neurology* 1980; 30:240–244.

Weinshenker BG, Penman M, Bass B, Ebers GC, Rice GPA. A double-blind, randomized, crossover trial of pemoline in fatigue associated with multiple sclerosis. *Neurology* 1992; 42:1468–1471.

Young RR (supplement editor). Role of tizanidine in the treatment of spasticity. *Neurology* 1994, Suppl. 9.

CHAPTER 13

Community Resources

Deborah P. Hertz, MPH,
and Nancy J. Holland, EdD, RN

Many resources are available for both the treating physician and the person with multiple sclerosis (MS). The information provided here is by no means complete, but it is a place to begin getting answers to your own clinical questions as well as the questions asked by your patients and their families.

This chapter is divided into two sections, resources for physicians about MS (professional organizations and professional education opportunities) and resources for people with MS and their families.

RESOURCES FOR PHYSICIANS ABOUT MS

American Academy of Neurology (AAN)
1080 Montreal Avenue
St. Paul, MN 55116-2325
Tel: (612) 695-1940
Fax: (612) 695-2791
Web site: www.aan.com

Mission: The AAN is a medical specialty society established to advance the art and science of neurology, and thereby promote the best possible care for patients with neurologic disorders by:

⊃ Ensuring appropriate access to neurologic care

⊃ Supporting and advocating an environment that ensures ethical, high quality neurologic care

⊃ Providing excellence in professional education through diverse programs in both the clinical aspects of neurology and the basic neurosciences

⊃ Supporting clinical and basic research in the neurosciences and related fields

In 1997 the AAN formed a section on MS. Its purpose is to further patient care, research, and teaching about MS. The section implements seminars, publications, presentations at scientific sessions of the AAN, and other events that encourage an increased level of interest in MS.

The Academy is developing a targeted educational series on MS, through a grant from the National Multiple Sclerosis Society's Clinical Programs Department.

Consortium of Multiple Sclerosis Centers (CMSC)
c/o Gimbel MS Center at Holy Name Hospital
718 Teaneck Road
Teaneck, New Jersey 07666
Tel: (201) 837-0727
Fax: (201) 837-8504
Web site: www.mscares.org

Mission: The mission of the Consortium is to disseminate information to clinicians, increase resources and opportunities for research, and advance the standard of care for people with MS.

The CMSC was established in 1986 as a multidisciplinary organization, bringing together professionals from the United States and Canada involved in MS patient care and research. Physicians, rehabilitation specialists, psychologists and neuropsychologists, social workers, scientists, nurses, and administrators are all active members of the organization. The annual meeting offers Continuing Education Units for physicians, nurses, physical therapists, speech and language pathologists, and psychologists.

The Consortium sponsors the North American Research Consortium on MS (NARCOMS), developed to facilitate multicenter research in MS. The "International Journal of MS Care" is the official journal of the CMSC and Rehabilitation in MS (RIMS). It is a quarterly, peer-reviewed journal available exclusively on the Internet.

Multiple Sclerosis Council for Clinical Practice Guidelines
c/o Paralyzed Veterans of America
801 Eighteenth Street, NW
Washington, DC 20006
Tel: (202) 872-1300
Fax: (202) 331-1657
Web site: www.pva.org

The MS Council includes representatives from 22 organizations that have a strong commitment to the welfare of people with MS, including access to quality, state-of-the-art health care. The goal of this collaborative effort is the development, dissemination, implementation, and evaluation of clinical practice guidelines for the many aspects of MS care.

These clinical practice guidelines are primarily evidence-based management strategies, developed to assist health care professionals in clinical decision making. The two completed topics (urinary dysfunction and fatigue) take into account the wide range of patients, clinicians, and treatment settings. Disease and relapse management, spasticity, and vaccinations are anticipated to be completed by the end of 1999, and pain and pregnancy during 2000. All topics were developed by a panel of experts from various disciplines.

The process was initiated in 1995 by the Consortium of MS Centers, the National Multiple Sclerosis Society, and the American Academy of Neurology, and expanded in 1997 under the administrative auspices of Paralyzed Veterans of America (PVA). Financial support for this process is provided by the PVA

Copies of the guidelines are available free of charge by calling the distribution center directly at 888-860-7244 or downloading a form from the PVA web site.

National Multiple Sclerosis Society
733 Third Avenue
New York, New York 10017
Tel: (212) 986-3240 or 1-800-FIGHT-MS
Fax: (212) 986-7981
Web site: www.nmss.org

Mission: To end the devastating effects of multiple sclerosis.

The National Multiple Sclerosis Society (NMSS) is the only nonprofit organization that supports national and international research (both basic and health services) into the prevention, cure, and treatment of MS. Equally important, the NMSS provides information about MS to people with MS, their families, health care professionals, and the public, and implements support programs for people with MS and their families, through a nation-wide network.

• One strategy the NMSS employs to improve the quality of heath care available to individuals with MS is the provision of continuing education programs for health care professionals. The Clinical Programs Department maintains a speakers' bureau and supports professional education pro-grams nationwide.

• The Americas Committee for Treatment and Research in Multiple Sclerosis (ACTRIMS) symposium, in collaboration with the NMSS and the MS Society of Canada, targets basic scientists with research interests in MS, clinical investigators in MS, and interested clinicians with an active practice focused on MS. Meetings are held in conjunction with the American Neu-rological Association's annual conference.

• The NMSS has more than 100 affiliations with MS facilities across the United States. The affiliation creates a collaborative approach to more effectively improve the quality of health care for people with MS by enhanc-ing both the NMSS and clinical facility's ability to reach people with MS in a given geographic area and to provide more comprehensive services. The NMSS affiliation process is *not* a certification process. It does, however, demonstrate the NMSS commitment to improving the lives of people with MS by working in close collaboration with the health care community. The list of affiliations is on the NMSS web site and can also be obtained by requesting a copy from your local chapter. Call 1-800-FIGHT-MS or the Clinical Programs Department at the home office at (212) 476-0456.

• The Research Department and the Clinical Programs Department regularly disseminate updates dealing both with current research topics and clinical issues. These can be obtained from the local chapters and divi-sions by calling 1-800-FIGHT-MS.

• *Consensus Statement:* For the first time, the medical advisors of the NMSS moved beyond the provision of information to the establishment of a recommendation relative to therapy. The consensus statement advises early intervention with one of the disease-modifying agents currently approved for use in MS by the Food and Drug Administration (FDA). An impetus for the development of this consensus statement was to facilitate access to therapies for disease management. The experience of MS experts as well as the data from clinical trials has shown that all three drugs offer benefits to people with relapsing-remitting MS. The evidence that permanent damage to axons is associated with MS, in addition to the destruction of myelin sheath, also suggests the importance of early inter-vention.

• Each NMSS chapter and division has a Clinical Advisory Committee comprised of community health professionals with expertise in MS. The committee advises chapters and divisions on programs with medical and health content to ensure that all information is current and accurate. The committee is also involved with the implementation of professional education programs administered locally. Members of the committee are potential resources to answer clinical questions about MS.

SELECTED BIBLIOGRAPHY

Textbooks

Burks JS, Johnson KP (eds.). *Multiple Sclerosis: Diagnosis, Medical Management, and Rehabilitation.* New York: Demos Medical Publishing, Inc., 2000 (in press).

Cook SD, ed. *Handbook of Multiple Sclerosis,* 2nd edition. New York: Marcel Dekker, Inc., 1996.

Goodkin DE, Rudick RA (eds.). *Multiple Sclerosis: Advances in Clinical Trial Design, Treatment and Future Perspectives.* London: Springer, 1996.

Paty DW, Ebers GC (eds.). *Multiple Sclerosis.* Philadelphia: F.A. Davis Company, 1998.

Raine CS, McFarland HF, Tourtellotte WW (eds.). *Multiple Sclerosis: Clinical and Pathogenic Basis.* London: Chapman & Hall, 1997.

Schapiro RT. *Symptom Management in Multiple Sclerosis,* 3rd edition. New York: Demos, 1998.

Sibley WA. *Therapeutic Claims in Multiple Sclerosis,* 4th edition. New York, Demos, 1996.

Thompson AF, Polman C, Hohlfeld R (eds.). *Multiple Sclerosis, Clinical Challenges and Controversies.* London: Martin Dunitz, 1997.

Periodicals

"Multiple Sclerosis, Clinical and Laboratory Research." Published by Stockton Press, a division of Macmillan press Ltd.

"MS Management." Published by the International Federation of Multiple Sclerosis Societies, 10 Heddon Street, London W1R 7LJ, England.

COMMUNITY RESOURCES FOR PEOPLE WITH MS AND THEIR FAMILIES

National Multiple Sclerosis Society
733 Third Avenue
New York, New York 10017
Tel: (212) 986-3240 or 1-800-FIGHT-MS

Mission: To end the devastating effects of MS.

The National Multiple Sclerosis Society (NMSS) provides education, emotional support, and a variety of other programs to people with MS, members of their families, and to the public, through a network of 138 chapters, branches, and divisions across the United States. The local chapters and divisions can be reached by calling 1-800-FIGHT-MS.

Programs offered by the NMSS are designed to help people with MS learn about health issues and maintain their independence while providing emotional support. Each chapter or division offers programs for people newly diagnosed, information and referral, a quarterly newsletter, a lending library with current books and videos on MS, support groups (self-help groups), and other educational programs and advocacy.

Information about the disease is the first and most frequent request the NMSS receives from people with MS. The NMSS has developed more than 40 publications, several of which have been translated into Spanish. The topics covered include diagnosis, symptoms, living well, family issues, emotional issues, employment, exercise, and more. Chapters also have networks of support groups, led by trained volunteers, and many chapters offer one-on-one peer counseling. Referrals are made to physicians, rehabilitation specialists, home care agencies, long-term care options, psychologists and other professionals knowledgeable about MS, accessible transportation, and recreational opportunities.

Multiple Sclerosis Society of Canada
200 Bloor Street East, Suite 1000
Toronto, Ontario M4W 3P9, Canada
Tel: (416) 922-6065
In Canada: 1-800-268-7582
Web site: www.mssoc.ca

Mission: To be a leader in finding a cure for multiple sclerosis and enabling people affected by MS to enhance their quality of life.

The Multiple Sclerosis Society of Canada has seven regional divisions and more than 130 chapters throughout Canada. They fund medical research programs, promote public education, and produce publications in both English and French.

The organization provides information on a wide variety of topics, including treatment, research, and social services through a database of articles, called "ASK MS Information System."

Well Spouse Foundation
P.O. Box 801
New York, New York 10023

Tel: (212) 685-8815
    (800) 838-0879
Fax: (212) 685-8676
Web site: www.wellspouse.org

The Well Spouse Foundation is a national not-for-profit membership organization that offers an emotional support network for significant others of a chronically ill partner. Services provided include advocacy for home health and long-term care, peer support, and a newsletter.

Centers for Independent Living

Centers for Independent Living (CIL) exist in every state and are supported by state funds through the Department of Human Services. They are community-based, not-for-profit, nonresidential organizations that serve people with disabilities. The CILs provide programs and services that promote independent living, although, there is variability in the specific programs offered at each center.

The *Directory of Independent Living Centers and Related Organizations* is a publication of the ILRU Research Training Center on Independent Living at TIRR. A copy of the directory can be obtained by calling (713) 520-0232.

Vocational Rehabilitation (VR)

Vocational rehabilitation programs are funded in every state in the United States by the Rehabilitation Services Administration under the U.S. Department of Education. Vocational rehabilitation services are meant to enable individuals to maximize employment opportunities, self-sufficiency, independence, and integration into the community. Services vary among states but must include:

➲ Assessment to determine eligibility and needs

➲ Counseling, guidance, and job placement services to maintain, regain, or advance in employment

➲ Vocational and other training, including higher education and the purchase of tools, materials, and books

➲ Rehabilitation technology services, including vehicular modification

➲ Supported employment

➲ Occupational licenses, tools, equipment, initial stocks and supplies

➲ Personal assistance services while receiving VR services

➲ Transportation, including van purchase or repair

➲ Interpreter services for individuals who are deaf and readers for individuals who are blind

➲ Telecommunications and other technologic aids and devices

➲ Physical or mental restoration to reduce or eliminate impediments to employment

➲ Maintenance for additional costs incurred during rehabilitation

The VR program in each state can be an important resource for people with MS.

Resources for Veterans

Department of Veterans Affairs (VA)
810 Vermont Avenue, NW
Washington, DC 20420
Tel: (202) 273-5400
Web site: www.va.gov

The VA medical system has MS specialty clinics throughout the country. Most exist within neurology departments, but some are located within physiatry (physical medicine and rehabilitation) departments.

The extent to which a veteran can access MS-specific benefits is based on whether the diagnosis is considered "service-connected" or "nonservice-connected." (A case is considered service-connected if there is documented evidence of initial symptoms within seven years of discharge.)

VA resources include medical management, rehabilitation, home modification, mobility aides and other equipment (i.e., exercise), transportation, and home care.

Other Veterans Groups

Many nonprofit organizations provide free benefits such as counseling and can help veterans navigate through the VA system. Some also advocate for benefits and provide other services not available through the VA. Besides providing representation for veterans, some provide nonmedical services.

Paralyzed Veterans of American (PVA)
801 Eighteenth Street, N.W.
Washington, DC 20006
Tel: (202) 872-1300
Web site: www.pva.org

Eastern Paralyzed Veterans Association (EPVA), the largest chapter of PVA, covers New Jersey, New York, Pennsylvania, and parts of Connecticut. EPVA has a program that provides members with a free home assessment to improve accessibility and develop modifications. It also sponsors the "MS Quarterly Report," which is published in cooperation with the NMSS. It is distributed to veterans at no charge and is available to nonveterans on a subscription basis.

Eastern Paralyzed Veterans Association
Headquarters
75-20 Astoria Boulevard
Jackson Heights, NY 11370-1177
Tel: (718) 803-EPVA or (800) 444-0120
Web site: www.epva.org

Home Care

A home care nurse can assist in the medical management of the person with MS in a variety of ways, including:

- ⊃ Administration of IV steroids for relapses
- ⊃ Intermittent catheterization and other bladder and bowel management
- ⊃ Teaching self-injection to the person with MS and/or a family member when a disease-modifying agent is initiated
- ⊃ Evaluation and treatment of decubitus ulcers
- ⊃ Management of indwelling catheters
- ⊃ Health screening such as blood pressure checks, wellness education, and education about MS

Visiting nurse associations, public health agencies, and private home care agencies offer both skilled nurses and personal care assistants, and frequently have other professionals, such as physical and occupational therapists and social workers, available for home visits.

SELECTED BIBLIOGRAPHY

Numerous publications are available to assist people with MS and their families. Many can be borrowed through the lending libraries of the local NMSS chapter.

Holland NJ, Murray TJ, Reingold SC. *Multiple Sclerosis: A Guide for the Newly Diagnosed.* New York: Demos Medical Publishing, 1996.

Holland NJ, Halper J (eds.). *Multiple Sclerosis: A Self-Care Guide to Wellness.* Washington, DC: Paralyzed Veterans of America, 1998.

Kalb R. *Multiple Sclerosis: A Guide for Families.* New York: Demos Medical Publishing, 1998.

Kalb R. *Multiple Sclerosis: The Questions You Have—The Answers You Need.* New York: Demos Medical Publishing, 1996.

Kraft GH, Catanzaro M. *Living with Multiple Sclerosis: A Wellness Approach.* New York: Demos Medical Publishing, 1996.

Perkins L, Perkins S. *Multiple Sclerosis: Your Legal; Rights,* 2nd edition. New York: Demos Medical Publishing (in press).

Peterman Schwarz S. *300 Tips for Making Life with Multiple Sclerosis Easier.* New York: Demos Medical Publishing, 1999.

Schapiro RT. *Symptom Management in Multiple Sclerosis,* 3rd edition. New York: Demos Medical Publishing, 1998.

"MS Quarterly Report." Published by the Eastern Paralyzed Veterans Association and the National Multiple Sclerosis Society. Copies are available free to veterans and at minimal charge to nonveterans through Demos Medical Publishing.

Information about the above titles may be obtained from Demos Medical Publishing, 386 Park Avenue South, New York, NY 10016, (800) 532-8663, info@demospub.com

Books About Personal Experiences

Burnfield A. *Multiple Sclerosis: A Personal Exploration,* 2nd edition. London: Souvenir Press, 1996

Koplowitz, Z. *The Winning Spirit: Life Lessons Learned in Last Place.* New York: Doubleday, 1997.

MacFarlane Burstein. *Legwork: An Inspiring Journey Through a Chronic Illness.* New York: Charles Scribner's Sons, 1994.

Medications Commonly Used in Multiple Sclerosis

The information sheets are intended as a patient's guide to drugs commonly used in the treatment and management of multiple sclerosis. They describe the ways in which each medication is most often prescribed in MS, as well as precautions to be noted and the side effects that may occur with their use. Those side effects that could possibly be confused with symptoms of multiple sclerosis are marked with an asterisk.

The information contained in these sheets will help your patients to be more informed about the medications they are taking and therefore more able to discuss their questions and concerns with their physician. This information should never be used as a substitute for professional instructions and recommendations.

The following guidelines will help your patients to manage their medication regime:

➲ Make sure that your physician knows your medical history, including all medical conditions for which you are currently being treated and any allergies you have.

➲ Tell your physician if you are breast-feeding, currently pregnant, or planning to become pregnant in the near future.

---

*Reprinted with permission of the publisher from *Multiple Sclerosis: The Questions You Have— The Answers You Need* edited by Rosalind C. Kalb. New York: Demos Vermande, 1996.

➲ Make a list of all of the drugs you are currently taking—including both prescription and over-the-counter medications—and provide your physician with a copy for your medical chart.

➲ Take your medications only as your physician prescribes them for you. If you have questions about the recommended dosage, ask your physician.

➲ Unless otherwise instructed, store medications in a cool, dry place; exposure to heat or moisture may cause the medication to break down. Liquid medications that are stored in the refrigerator should not be allowed to freeze.

➲ Unless otherwise directed by your physician or pharmacist, the general instructions concerning a missed dose of medication are as follows: if you miss a dose, take it as soon as possible. However, if it is almost time for your next dose, skip the one you missed and go back to the regular dosing schedule. Do not double dose.

➲ Keep all medications out of the reach of children.

Index of Medications

Prescription

Amantadine
Amitriptyline
Baclofen
Carbamazepine
Ciprofloxacin
Clonazepam
Desmopressin
Diazepam
Fluoxetine
Imipramine
Interferon beta-1a
Interferon beta-1b
Meclizine

Methenamine
Methylprednisolone
Oxybutynin
Papaverine
Paroxetine
Pemoline
Phenazopyridine
Phenytoin
Prednisone
Propantheline bromide
Sertraline
Sulfamethoxazole and
    trimethoprim combination

Non-Prescription
(Over-the-Counter)

Bisacodyl (Dulcolax)—
  tablet or suppository
Docusate (Colace)
Docusate mini enema
  (Therevac Plus)
Glycerin suppository
Magnesium hydroxide
  (Phillips' Milk of Magnesia)

Mineral oil
Psyllium hydrophilic
  mucilloid (Metamucil)
Sodium phosphate
  (Fleet Enema)

Chemical Name: Amantadine (a-**man**-ta-deen)

Brand Name: Symmetrel (U.S. and Canada)

Generic Available: Yes (U.S.)

Description: Amantadine is an antiviral medication used to prevent or treat certain influenza infections; it is also given as an adjunct for the treatment of Parkinson's disease. It has been demonstrated that this medication, through some unknown mechanism, is sometimes effective in relieving fatigue in multiple sclerosis.

Proper Usage

⊃ The usual dosage for the management of fatigue in MS is 100 to 200 mg daily, taken in the earlier part of the day in order to avoid sleep disturbance. Doses in excess of 300 mg daily usually cause livedo reticularis, a blotchy discoloration of the skin of the legs.

Precautions

The precautions listed here pertain to the use of this medication as an antiviral or Parkinson's disease treatment. There are no reports at this time concerning the precautions in the use of the drug to treat fatigue in multiple sclerosis.

⊃ Drinking alcoholic beverages while taking this medication may cause increased side effects such as circulation problems, dizziness, lightheadedness, fainting, or confusion. Do not drink alcohol while taking this medication.

⊃ This medication may cause some people to become dizzy, confused, or lightheaded, or to have blurred vision or trouble concentrating.

⊃ Amantadine may cause dryness of the mouth and throat. If your mouth continues to feel dry for more than two weeks, check with your physician or dentist since continuing dryness may increase the risk of dental disease.

⊃ This medication may cause purplish red, net-like, blotchy spots on the skin. This problem occurs more often in females and usually occurs on the legs and/or feet after amantadine has been taken regularly for a month or more. The blotchy spots usually go away within two to twelve weeks after you stop taking the medication.

⊃ Studies of the effects of amantadine in pregnancy have not been done in humans. Studies in some animals have shown that amantadine is harmful to the fetus and causes birth defects.

⊃ Amantadine passes into breast milk. However, the effect of amantadine in newborn babies and infants is not known.

Possible Side Effects

The side effects listed here pertain to the use of amantadine as an antiviral or Parkinson's disease treatment. There are no reports at the present time of the side effects associated with the use of this drug in the treatment of MS-related fatigue.

➲ Side effects that may go away as your body adjusts to the medication and do not require medical attention unless they continue or are bothersome: difficulty concentrating; dizziness; headache; irritability; loss of appetite; nausea; nervousness; purplish red, net-like, blotchy spots on skin; trouble sleeping or nightmares; constipation*; dryness of the mouth; vomiting.

➲ Rare side effects that should be reported as soon as possible to your physician: blurred vision*; confusion; difficult urination*; fainting; hallucinations; convulsions; unusual difficulty in coordination*; irritation and swelling of the eye; mental depression; skin rash; swelling of feet or lower legs; unexplained shortness of breath.

*Since it may be difficult to distinguish between certain common symptoms of MS and some side effects of amantadine, be sure to consult your health care professional if an abrupt change of this type continues for more than a few days.

Chemical Name: Amitriptyline (a-mee-**trip**-ti-leen)

Brand Name: Elavil (U.S. and Canada)

Generic Available: Yes (U.S. and Canada)

Description: Amitriptyline is a tricyclic antidepressant used to treat mental depression. In multiple sclerosis, it is frequently used to treat painful paresthesias in the arms and legs (e.g., burning sensations, pins and needles, stabbing pains) caused by damage to the pain regulating pathways of the brain and spinal cord.

Note: Other tricyclic antidepressants are also used for the management of neurologic pain symptoms. Clomipramine (Anafranil—U.S. and Canada), desipramine (Norpramin—U.S. and Canada), doxepin (Sinequan—U.S. and Canada), imipramine (Tofranil—U.S. and Canada), nortriptyline (Pamelor—U.S.; Aventyl—Canada), trimipramine (U.S. and Canada). While each of these medications is given in different dosage levels, the precautions and side effects listed for amitriptyline apply to these other tricyclic medications as well.

Precautions

⊃ Amitriptyline adds to the effects of alcohol and other central nervous system depressants (e.g., antihistamines, sedatives, tranquilizers, prescription pain medications, seizure medications, muscle relaxants, sleeping medications), possibly causing drowsiness. Be sure that your physician knows if you are taking these or other medications.

⊃ This medication causes dryness of the mouth. Because continuing dryness of the mouth may increase the risk of dental disease, alert your dentist that you are taking amitriptyline.

⊃ This medication may cause your skin to be more sensitive to sunlight than it is normally. Even brief exposure to sunlight may cause a skin rash, itching, redness or other discoloration of the skin, or severe sunburn.

⊃ This medication may affect blood sugar levels of diabetic individuals. If you notice a change in the results of your blood or urine sugar tests, check with your physician.

⊃ Do not stop taking this medication without consulting your physician. The physician may want you to reduce the amount you are taking gradually in order to reduce the possibility of withdrawal symptoms such as headache, nausea, and/or an overall feeling of discomfort.

⊃ Studies of amitriptyline have not been done in pregnant women. There have been reports of newborns suffering from muscle spasms and heart, breathing, and urinary problems when their mothers had taken tricyclic antidepressants immediately before delivery. Studies in animals have indicated the possibility of unwanted effects in the fetus.

➲ Tricyclics pass into breast milk. Only doxepin (Sinequan) has been reported to cause drowsiness in the nursing baby.

Possible Side Effects

➲ Side effects that may go away as your body adjusts to the medication and do not require medical attention unless they continue for more than two weeks or are bothersome: dryness of mouth; constipation*; increased appetite and weight gain; dizziness; drowsiness*; decreased sexual ability*; headache; nausea; unusual tiredness or weakness*; unpleasant taste; diarrhea; heartburn; increased sweating; vomiting.

➲ Uncommon side effects that should be reported to your physician as soon as possible: blurred vision*; confusion or delirium; difficulty speaking or swallowing*; eye pain*; fainting; hallucinations; loss of balance control*; nervousness or restlessness; problems urinating*; shakiness or trembling; stiffness of arms and legs*.

➲ Rare side effects that should be reported to your physician as soon as possible: anxiety; breast enlargement in males and females; hair loss; inappropriate secretion of milk in females; increased sensitivity to sunlight; irritability; muscle twitching; red or brownish spots on the skin; buzzing or other unexplained sounds in the ears; skin rash, itching; sore throat and fever; swelling of face and tongue; weakness*; yellow skin.

➲ Symptoms of acute overdose: confusion; convulsions; severe drowsiness*; enlarged pupils; unusual heartbeat; fever; hallucinations; restlessness and agitation; shortness of breath; unusual tiredness or weakness; vomiting.

*Since it may be difficult to distinguish between certain common symptoms of MS and some side effects of amitriptyline, be sure to consult your health care professional if an abrupt change of this type occurs.

Chemical Name: Baclofen (**bak**-loe-fen)

Brand Name: Lioresal (U.S. and Canada)

Generic Available: Yes (U.S. and Canada)

Description: Baclofen acts on the central nervous system to relieve spasms, cramping, and tightness of muscles caused by spasticity in multiple sclerosis. It is usually administered orally in pill form. Recently, an intrathecal delivery system (via a surgically implanted pump) has been approved for those individuals with significant spasticity who cannot tolerate a sufficiently high dose of the oral form of the medication.

Proper Usage

⊃ People with MS are usually started on an initial dose of 5 mg every six to eight hours. If necessary, the amount is increased by 5 mg per dose every five days until symptoms improve. The goal of treatment is to find a dosage level that relieves spasticity without causing excessive weakness or fatigue. The effective dose may vary from 15 mg to 160 mg per day or more.

Precautions

⊃ If you are taking more than 30 mg daily, do not stop taking this medication suddenly. Stopping high doses of this medication abruptly can cause convulsions, hallucinations, increases in muscle spasms or cramping, mental changes, or unusual nervousness or restlessness. Consult your physician about how to reduce the dosage gradually before stopping the medication completely.

⊃ This drug adds to the effects of alcohol and other CNS depressants (such as antihistamines, sedatives, tranquilizers, prescription pain medications, seizure medications, other muscle relaxants), possibly causing drowsiness. Be sure that your physician knows if you are taking these or other medications.

⊃ Studies of birth defects with baclofen have not been done with humans. Studies in animals have shown that baclofen, when given in doses several times higher than the amount given to humans, increases the chance of hernias, incomplete or slow development of bones in the fetus, and lower birth weight.

⊃ Baclofen passes into the breast milk of nursing mothers but has not been reported to cause problems in nursing infants.

Possible Side Effects

⊃ Side effects that typically go away as your body adjusts to the medication and do not require medical attention unless they continue for several weeks or are bothersome: drowsiness or unusual tiredness*; increased weakness*; dizziness or lightheadedness; confusion; unusual constipation*; new or unusual bladder symptoms*; trouble sleeping; unusual unsteadiness or clumsiness*.

⊃ Unusual side effects that require immediate medical attention: fainting; hallucinations; severe mood changes; skin rash or itching.

⊃ Symptoms of overdose: sudden onset of blurred or double vision*; convulsions; shortness of breath or troubled breathing; vomiting.

*Since it may be difficult to distinguish between certain common symptoms of MS and some side effects of baclofen, be sure to consult your health care professional if an abrupt change of this type occurs.

Chemical Name: Bisacodyl (bis-a-**koe**-dill)

Brand Name: Dulcolax—tablet or suppository (U.S.); Bisacolax—tablet or suppository (Canada)

Generic Available: Yes (U.S. and Canada)

Description: Bisacodyl is an over-the-counter stimulant laxative that can be used in either oral or suppository form. Stimulant laxatives encourage bowel movements by increasing the muscle contractions in the intestinal wall that propel the stool mass. Although stimulant laxatives are popular for self-treatment, they are more likely to cause side effects than other types of laxatives.

Proper Usage

⊃ Laxatives are to be used to provide short-term relief only, unless otherwise directed by the nurse or physician who is helping you to manage your bowel symptoms. A regimen that includes a healthy diet containing roughage (whole grain breads and cereals, bran, fruit, and green, leafy vegetables), six to eight full glasses of liquids each day, and some form of daily exercise is most important in stimulating healthy bowel function.

⊃ If your physician has recommended this laxative for management of constipation, follow his or her recommendations for its use. If you are treating yourself for constipation, follow the directions on the package insert.

⊃ The tablet form of this laxative is usually taken on an empty stomach in order to speed results. The tablets are coated to allow them to work properly without causing stomach irritation or upset. Do not chew or crush the tablets or take them within an hour of drinking milk or taking an antacid.

⊃ A bedtime dose usually produces results the following morning. Be sure to consult your physician if you experience problems or do not get relief within a week.

Precautions

⊃ Do not take any laxative if you have signs of appendicitis or inflamed bowel (e.g., stomach or lower abdominal pain, cramping, bloating, soreness, nausea, or vomiting). Check with your physician as soon as possible.

⊃ Do not take any laxative for more than one week unless you have been told to do so by your physician. Many people tend to overuse laxatives, which often leads to dependence on the laxative action to produce a bowel movement. Discuss the use of laxatives with your health care professional in order to ensure that the laxative is used effectively as part of a comprehensive, healthy bowel management regimen.

⊃ Do not take any laxative within two hours of taking other medication because the desired effectiveness of the other medication may be reduced.

⊃ If you are pregnant, discuss with your physician the most appropriate type of laxative for you to use.

⊃ Some laxatives pass into breast milk. Although it is unlikely to cause problems for a nursing infant, be sure to let your physician know if you are using a laxative and breast-feeding at the same time.

Possible Side Effects

⊃ Side effects that may go away as your body adjusts to the medication and do not require medical attention unless they persist or are bothersome: belching; cramping; diarrhea; nausea.

⊃ Unusual side effects that should be reported to your physician as soon as possible: confusion; irregular heartbeat; muscle cramps; skin rash, unusual tiredness or weakness.

Chemical Name: Carbamazepine (kar-ba-**maz**-e-peen)

Brand Name: Tegretol (U.S. and Canada)

Generic Available: Yes (U.S.)

Description: Carbamazepine is used to relieve shock-like pain, such as the facial pain caused by trigeminal neuralgia (tic douloureux).

Proper Usage

⊃ It is very important that you take this medicine exactly as directed by your physician in order to obtain the best results and lessen the chance of serious side effects.

⊃ Carbamazepine is not an ordinary pain reliever. It should be used only when your physician prescribes it for certain types of pain. Do not take this medication for other aches or pains.

⊃ If you miss a dose of this medication, take it as soon as possible. If it is almost time for your next dose, skip the missed dose and go back to your regular dosing schedule. Do not double dose. If you miss more than one dose in a day, check with your physician.

⊃ It is very important that your physician check your progress at regular intervals. Your physician may want to have certain tests done to see if you are receiving the correct amount of medication or to check for certain side effects of which you might be unaware.

Precautions

⊃ Carbamazepine adds to the effects of alcohol and other central nervous system depressants that may cause drowsiness (e.g., antihistamines, sedatives, tranquilizers, prescription pain medications, seizure medications, muscle relaxants). Be sure that your physician knows if you are taking these or other medications.

⊃ Some people who take carbamazepine may become more sensitive to sunlight than they are normally. Exposure to sunlight, even for brief periods of time, may cause a skin rash, itching, redness or other discoloration of the skin, or severe sunburn.

⊃ Oral contraceptives (birth control pills) that contain estrogen may not work properly while you are taking carbamazepine. You should use an additional or alternative form of birth control while taking this drug.

⊃ Carbamazepine affects the urine sugar levels of diabetic patients. If you notice a change in the results of your urine sugar tests, check with your physician.

⊃ Before having any medical tests or any kind of surgical, dental, or emergency treatment, be sure to let the health care professional know that you are taking this medication.

⊃ Carbamazepine has not been studied in pregnant women. There have been reports of babies having low birth weight, small head size, skull and facial defects, underdeveloped fingernails, and delays in growth when their mothers had taken carbamazepine in high doses during pregnancy. Studies in animals have shown that carbamazepine causes birth defects when given in large doses.

⊃ Carbamazepine passes into breast milk, and the baby may receive enough of it to cause unwanted effects. In animal studies, carbamazepine has affected the growth and appearance of nursing babies.

Possible Side Effects

⊃ Side effects that typically go away as your body adjusts to the medication and do not require medical attention unless they continue for several weeks or are bothersome: clumsiness or unsteadiness*; mild dizziness*; mild drowsiness*; lightheadedness; mild nausea or vomiting; aching joints or muscles; constipation*; diarrhea; dryness of mouth; skin sensitivity to sunlight; irritation of mouth or tongue; loss of appetite; loss of hair; muscle or abdominal cramps; sexual problems in males*.

⊃ Check with your physician as soon as possible if any of the following side effects occur: blurred or double vision*; confusion; agitation; severe diarrhea, nausea, or vomiting; skin rash or hives; unusual drowsiness; chest pain; difficulty speaking or slurred speech*; fainting; frequent urination*; unusual heartbeat; mental depression or other mood or emotional changes; unusual numbness, tingling, pain, or weakness in hands or feet*; ringing or buzzing in ears; sudden decrease in urination; swelling of face, hands, feet, or lower legs; trembling; uncontrolled body movements; visual hallucinations.

⊃ Check with your physician immediately if any of the following occur: black tarry stools or blood in urine or stools; bone or joint pain; cough or hoarseness; darkening of urine; nosebleeds or other unusual bleeding or bruising; painful or difficult urination; tenderness, swelling, or bluish color in leg or foot; pale stools; pinpoint red spots on skin; shortness of breath or cough; sores, ulcers, or white spots on lips or in the mouth; sore throat, chills, and fever; swollen glands; unusual tiredness or weakness*; wheezing, tightness in chest; yellow eyes or skin.

⊃ Symptoms of overdose that require immediate attention: unusual clumsiness or unsteadiness*; severe dizziness or fainting; fast or irregular heartbeat; unusually high or low blood pressure; irregular or shallow breathing; severe nausea or vomiting; trembling, twitching, and abnormal body movements.

*Since it may be difficult to distinguish between certain common symptoms of MS and some side effects of carbamazepine, be sure to consult your health care professional if an abrupt change of this type occurs.

Chemical Name: Ciprofloxacin (sip-roe-**flox**-a-sin) combination

Brand Name: Cipro (U.S. and Canada)

Generic Available: No

Description: Ciprofloxacin is one of a group of antibiotics (fluoro-quinolones) used to kill bacterial infection in many parts of the body. It is used in multiple sclerosis primarily to treat urinary tract infections.

Proper Usage

- ⊃ This medication is best taken with a full glass (eight ounces) of water. Additional water should be taken each day to help prevent some unwanted effects.
- ⊃ Ciprofloxacin may be taken with meals or on an empty stomach.
- ⊃ Finish the full course of treatment prescribed by your physician. Even if your symptoms disappear after a few days, stopping this medication prematurely may result in a return of the symptoms.
- ⊃ This medication works most effectively when it is maintained at a constant level in your blood or urine. To help keep the amount constant, do not miss a dose. It is best to take the doses at evenly spaced times during the day and night.

Precautions

- ⊃ This medication may cause some people to become dizzy, light-headed, drowsy, or less alert.
- ⊃ If you are taking antacids that contain aluminum or magnesium, be sure to take them at least two hours before or after you take ciprofloxacin. These antacids may prevent the ciprofloxacin from working properly.
- ⊃ This medication may cause your skin to become more sensitive to sunlight. Stay out of direct sunlight during the midday hours, wear protective clothing, and apply a sun block product that has a skin protection factor (SPF) of at least 15.
- ⊃ Studies of birth defects have not been done in humans. This medication is not recommended during pregnancy since antibiotics of this type have been reported to cause bone development problems in young animals.
- ⊃ Some of the antibiotics in this group are known to pass into human breast milk. Since they have been reported to cause bone development problems in young animals, breast-feeding is not recommended during treatment with this medication.

Possible Side Effects

➲ Side effects that may go away as your body adjusts to the medication and do not require medical attention unless they continue or are bothersome: abdominal or stomach pain; diarrhea; dizziness; drowsiness*; headache; lightheadedness; nausea or vomiting; nervousness; trouble sleeping.

➲ Rare side effects that should be reported to your physician immediately: agitation; confusion; fever; hallucinations; peeling of the skin; shakiness or tremors*; shortness of breath; skin rash; itching; swelling of face or neck.

*Since it may be difficult to distinguish between certain common symptoms of MS and some side effects of ciprofloxacin, be sure to consult your health care professional if an abrupt change of this type occurs.

Chemical Name: Clonazepam (kloe-**na**-ze-pam)

Brand Name: Klonopin (U.S.); Rivotril; Syn-Clonazepam (Canada)

Generic Available: No

Description: Clonazepam is a benzodiazepine that belongs to the group of medications called central nervous system depressants, which slow down the nervous system. Although clonazepam is used for a variety of medical conditions, it is used in multiple sclerosis primarily for the treatment of tremor, pain, and spasticity.

Proper Usage

⮱ Keep this medication out of the reach of children. An overdose of this medication may be especially dangerous for children.

Precautions

⮱ During the first few months taking clonazepam, your physician should check your progress at regular visits to make sure that this medicine does not cause unwanted effects.

⮱ Take this medication only as directed by your physician; do not increase the dose without a prescription to do so.

⮱ Clonazepam adds to the effects of alcohol and other central nervous system depressants (e.g., antihistamines, sedatives, tranquilizers, prescription pain medications, seizure medications, muscle relaxants, sleeping medications). Consult your physician before taking any of these CNS depressants while you are taking clonazepam. Taking an overdose of this medication or taking it with alcohol or other CNS depressants may lead to unconsciousness and possibly death.

⮱ Stopping this medication suddenly may cause withdrawal side effects. Reduce the amount gradually before stopping completely.

⮱ Clonazepam frequently causes people to become drowsy, dizzy, lightheaded, clumsy, or unsteady. Even if taken at bedtime, it may cause some people to feel drowsy or less alert on awakening.

⮱ Studies in animals have shown that clonazepam can cause birth defects or other problems, including death of the animal fetus.

⮱ Overuse of clonazepam during pregnancy may cause the baby to become dependent on it, leading to withdrawal side effects after birth. The use of clonazepam, especially during the last weeks of pregnancy, may cause breathing problems, muscle weakness, difficulty in feeding, and body temperature problems in the newborn infant.

➲ Clonazepam may pass into breast milk and cause drowsiness, slow heartbeat, shortness of breath, or troubled breathing in nursing babies.

Possible Side Effects

➲ Side effects that may go away during treatment as your body adjusts to the medication and do not require medical attention unless they continue for several weeks or are bothersome: drowsiness or tiredness; clumsiness or unsteadiness*; dizziness or lightheadedness; slurred speech*; abdominal cramps or pain; blurred vision or other changes in vision*; changes in sexual drive or performance*; gastrointestinal changes, including constipation* or diarrhea; dryness of mouth; fast or pounding heartbeat; muscle spasm*; trouble with urination*; trembling.

➲ Unusual side effects that should be discussed as soon as possible with your physician: behavior problems, including difficulty concentrating and outbursts of anger; confusion or mental depression; convulsions; hallucinations; low blood pressure; muscle weakness; skin rash or itching; sore throat, fever, chills; unusual bleeding or bruising; unusual excitement or irritability.

➲ Symptoms of overdose that require immediate emergency help: continuing confusion; severe drowsiness; shakiness; slowed heartbeat; shortness of breath; slow reflexes; continuing slurred speech*; staggering*; unusual severe weakness*.

*Since it may be difficult to distinguish between certain common symptoms of MS and some side effects of clonazepam, be sure to consult your health care professional if an abrupt change of this type occurs.

Chemical Name: Desmopressin (des-moe-**press**-in)

Brand Name: DDAVP Nasal Spray (U.S. and Canada)

Generic Available: No

Description: Desmopressin is a hormone used as a nasal spray. The hormone works on the kidneys to control frequent urination.

Proper Usage

⊃ Keep this medication in the refrigerator but do not allow it to freeze.

Precautions

⊃ Let your physician know if you have heart disease, blood vessel disease, or high blood pressure. Desmopressin can cause an increase in blood pressure.

⊃ Studies have not been done in pregnant women. It has been used before and during pregnancy to treat diabetes mellitus and has not been shown to cause birth defects.

⊃ Desmopressin passes into breast milk but has not been reported to cause problems in nursing infants.

Possible Side Effects

⊃ Side effects that typically go away as your body adjusts to the medication and do not require medical attention unless they continue for several weeks or are bothersome: runny or stuffy nose; abdominal or stomach cramps; flushing of the skin; headache; nausea; pain in the vulva.

⊃ Unusual side effects that require immediate medical attention: confusion; convulsions; unusual drowsiness*; continuing headache; rapid weight gain; markedly decreased urination.

*Since it may be difficult to distinguish between certain common symptoms of MS and some side effects of desmopressin, be sure to consult your health care professional if an abrupt change of this type occurs.

Chemical Name: Diazepam (dye-**az**-e-pam)

Brand Name: Valium (U.S. and Canada)

Generic Available: Yes (U.S.)

Description: Diazepam is a benzodiazepine that belongs to the group of medicines called central nervous system depressants, which slow down the nervous system. Although diazepam is used for a variety of medical conditions, it is used in multiple sclerosis primarily for the relief of muscle spasms and spasticity.

Proper Usage

⊃ Keep this medication out of the reach of children. An overdose of this medication may be especially dangerous for children.

Precautions

⊃ Your physician should check your progress at regular visits to make sure that this medication does not cause unwanted effects.

⊃ Take diazepam only as directed by your physician; do not increase the dose without a prescription to do so.

⊃ Diazepam adds to the effects of alcohol and other central nervous system depressants (e.g., antihistamines, sedatives, tranquilizers, prescription pain medications, seizure medications, muscle relaxants, sleeping medications). Consult your physician before taking any of these CNS depressants while you are taking diazepam. Taking an overdose of this medication or taking it with alcohol or other CNS depressants may lead to unconsciousness and possibly death.

⊃ Stopping this medication suddenly may cause withdrawal side effects. Reduce the amount gradually before stopping completely.

⊃ Diazepam may cause some people to become drowsy, dizzy, light-headed, clumsy, or unsteady. Even if taken at bedtime, it may cause some people to feel drowsy or less alert on awakening.

⊃ The use of diazepam during the first three months of pregnancy has been reported to increase the chance of birth defects.

⊃ Overuse of diazepam during pregnancy may cause the baby to become dependent on the medicine, leading to withdrawal side effects after birth. The use of diazepam, especially during the last weeks of pregnancy, may cause breathing problems, muscle weakness, difficulty in feeding, and body temperature problems in the newborn infant. When diazepam is given in high doses (especially by injection) within fifteen hours before delivery, it may cause breathing problems, muscle weakness, difficulty in feeding, and body temperature problems in the newborn infant.⊃ Diazepam may pass into breast milk and cause drowsiness, slow heartbeat, shortness of breath, or troubled breathing in nursing babies.

Possible Side Effects

⊃ Side effects that may go away during treatment as your body adjusts to the medication and do not require medical attention unless they continue for several weeks or are bothersome: clumsiness or unsteadiness*; dizziness or lightheadedness; slurred speech*; abdominal cramps or pain; blurred vision or other changes in vision*; changes in sexual drive or performance*; constipation*; diarrhea; dryness of mouth; fast or pounding heartbeat; muscle spasm*; trouble with urination*; trembling*; unusual tiredness or weakness*.

⊃ Unusual side effects that should be discussed with your physician as soon as possible: behavior problems, including difficulty concentrating and outbursts of anger; confusion or mental depression; convulsions; hallucinations; low blood pressure; muscle weakness*; skin rash or itching; sore throat, fever, chills; unusual bleeding or bruising; unusual excitement or irritability.

⊃ Symptoms of overdose that require immediate emergency help: continuing confusion; unusually severe drowsiness; shakiness; slowed heartbeat; shortness of breath; slow reflexes; continuing slurred speech; staggering; unusually severe weakness*.

*Since it may be difficult to distinguish between certain common symptoms of MS and some side effects of diazepam, be sure to consult your health care professional if an abrupt change of this type occurs.

Chemical Name: Docusate (**doe**-koo-sate)

Brand Name: Colace (U.S. and Canada)

Generic Available: Yes (U.S. and Canada)

Description: Docusate is an over-the-counter stool softener (emollient) that helps liquids to mix into dry, hardened stool, making the stool easier to pass.

Proper Usage

⊃ Laxatives are to be used to provide short-term relief only, unless otherwise directed by the nurse or physician who is helping you to manage your bowel symptoms. A regimen that includes a healthy diet containing roughage (whole grain breads and cereals, bran, fruit, and green, leafy vegetables), six to eight full glasses of liquids each day, and some form of daily exercise is most important in stimulating healthy bowel function.

⊃ If your physician has recommended this laxative for management of constipation, follow his or her recommendations for its use. If you are treating yourself for constipation, follow the directions on the package insert.

⊃ Results usually occur one to two days after the first dose; some individuals may not get results for three to five days. Be sure to consult your physician if you experience problems or do not get relief within a week.

Precautions

⊃ Do not take any type of laxative if you have signs of appendicitis or inflamed bowel (e.g., stomach or lower abdominal pain, cramping, bloating, soreness, nausea, or vomiting). Check with your physician as soon as possible.

⊃ Do not take any laxative for more than one week unless you have been told to do so by your physician. Many people tend to overuse laxatives, which often leads to dependence on the laxative action to produce a bowel movement. Discuss the use of laxatives with your health care professional in order to ensure that the laxative is used effectively as part of a comprehensive, healthy bowel management regimen.

⊃ Do not take mineral oil within two hours of taking docusate. The docusate may increase the amount of mineral oil that is absorbed by the body.

⊃ Do not take any laxative within two hours of taking another medication because the desired effectiveness of the other medication may be reduced.

⊃ If you are pregnant, discuss with your physician the most appropriate type of laxative for you to use.

⊃ Some laxatives pass into breast milk. Although it is unlikely to cause problems for a nursing infant, be sure to let your physician know if you are using a laxative and breast-feeding at the same time.

Possible Side Effects

⊃ Side effects that may go away as your body adjusts to the medication and do not require medical attention unless they persist or are bothersome: stomach and/or intestinal cramping.

⊃ Unusual side effect that should be reported to your physician as soon as possible: skin rash.

Chemical Name: Fluoxetine (floo-**ox**-uh-teen)

Brand Name: Prozac (U.S. and Canada)

Generic Available: No

Description: Fluoxetine is used to treat mental depression. It is also used occasionally to treat MS fatigue.

Proper Usage

⊃ This medication should be taken in the morning when used to treat depression because it can interfere with sleep. If it upsets your stomach, you may take it with food.

Precautions

⊃ It may take four to six weeks for you to feel the beneficial effects of this medication.

⊃ Your physician should monitor your progress at regularly scheduled visits in order to adjust the dose and help reduce any side effects.

⊃ There have been suggestions that the use of fluoxetine may be related to increased thoughts about suicide in a very small number of individuals. More study is needed to determine if the medicine causes this effect. If you have concerns about this, be sure to discuss them with your physician.

⊃ Fluoxetine adds to the effects of alcohol and other central nervous system depressants (e.g., antihistamines, sedatives, tranquilizers, sleeping medicine, prescription pain medicine, barbiturates, seizure medication, muscle relaxants). Be sure that your physician knows if you are taking these or any other medications.

⊃ This medication affects the blood sugar levels of diabetic individuals. Check with your physician if you notice any changes in your blood or urine sugar tests.

⊃ Dizziness or lightheadedness may occur, especially when you get up from a lying or sitting position. Change positions slowly to help alleviate this problem. If the problem continues or gets worse, consult your physician.

⊃ Fluoxetine may cause dryness of the mouth. If your mouth continues to feel dry for more than two weeks, check with your physician or dentist. Continuing dryness of the mouth may increase the chance of dental disease.

⊃ Studies have not been done in pregnant women. Fluoxetine has not been shown to cause birth defects or other problems in animal studies.

⊃ Fluoxetine passes into breast milk and may cause unwanted effects, such as vomiting, watery stools, crying, and sleep problems in nursing babies. You may want to discuss alternative medications with your physician.

Possible Side Effects

⊃ Side effects that may go away as your body adjusts to the medication and do not require medical attention unless they continue for several weeks or are bothersome: decreased sexual drive or ability*; anxiety and nervousness; diarrhea; drowsiness*; headache; trouble sleeping; abnormal dreams; change in vision*; chest pain; decreased appetite; decrease in concentration; dizziness; dry mouth; fast or irregular heartbeat; frequent urination*; menstrual pain; tiredness or weakness*; tremor*; vomiting.

⊃ Unusual side effects that should be discussed with your physician as soon as possible: chills or fever; joint or muscle pain; skin rash; hives or itching; trouble breathing.

⊃ Symptoms of overdose that require immediate medical attention: agitation and restlessness; convulsions; severe nausea and vomiting; unusual excitement.

*Since it may be difficult to distinguish between certain common symptoms of MS and some side effects of fluoxetine, be sure to consult your health care professional if an abrupt change of this type occurs.

Chemical Name: Gabapentin (**ga**-ba-pen-tin)

Brand Name: Neurontin

Generic Available: No

Description: Gabapentin is used to control some types of seizures in the treatment of epilepsy. In MS it is used for the control of dysesthetic pain (pain caused by an MS lesion) and the pain due to spasticity.

Proper Usage

⊃ Gabapentin may be taken with or without food. Wait two hours after taking an antacid.

⊃ If gabapentin is taken three times a day you should not allow more than 12 hours to elapse between any two doses.

Precautions

⊃ Gabapentin adds to the effects of alcohol and other central nervous system depressants.

⊃ Inform your physician or your dentist that you are taking gabapentin before taking any of the following: antihistamines; sedatives; tranquilizers; sleeping medicines; prescription pain medications; seizure medications; muscle relaxants; anesthetics (including dental).

⊃ You should not stop taking gabapentin suddenly. Stopping suddenly may cause seizures. Your physician may want to lower your dose gradually.

⊃ Tell your physician you are taking gabapentin before having any medical tests. Some test results may be affected.

⊃ Gabapentin may cause drowsiness, blurred or double vision, dizziness, or trouble thinking. Be sure you are familiar with the effects of this medication before driving or operating machinery.

⊃ Gabapentin has not been studied in pregnant women. Animal studies have shown possible bone or kidney problems in offspring.

⊃ It is not known whether gabapentin passes into breast milk. Women should consult their physician before breast-feeding.

Possible Side Effects

⊃ Side effects that usually go away as your body adjusts to the medication and do not require medical attention unless they last for more than two weeks or are bothersome: Common: blurred or double vision; dizziness; drowsiness; muscle ache; swelling of hand or lower extremities; tremor; unusual tiredness; weakness. Less common: diarrhea; dry mouth; frequent urination; headache; indigestion; low blood pressure; nausea; slurred speech; noise in the ears; trouble thinking; sleep difficulty; vomiting; weakness; weight gain.

⊃ Side effects that should be reported to your physician as soon as possible: clumsiness or unsteadiness; continuous uncontrolled eye movements; depression; mood changes; irritability; memory problems; fever or chills; hoarseness; lower back pain; painful or difficult urination.

⊃ Symptoms of overdose include double vision; severe diarrhea; dizziness; drowsiness; slurred speech.

Chemical Name: Glycerin (**gli**-ser-in)

Brand Name: Sani-Supp suppository (U.S.)

Generic Available: Yes (U.S. and Canada)

Description: A glycerin suppository is a hyperosmotic laxative that draws water into the bowel from surrounding body tissues. This water helps to soften the stool mass and promote bowel action.

Proper Usage

◑ Laxatives are to be used to provide short-term relief only, unless otherwise directed by the nurse or physician who is helping you to manage your bowel symptoms. A regimen that includes a healthy diet containing roughage (whole grain breads and cereals, bran, fruit, and green, leafy vegetables), six to eight full glasses of liquids each day, and some form of daily exercise is most important in stimulating healthy bowel function.

◑ If your physician has recommended this laxative for management of constipation, follow his or her recommendations for its use. If you are treating yourself for constipation, follow the directions on the package insert.

◑ If the suppository is too soft to insert, refrigerate it for thirty minutes or hold it under cold water before removing the foil wrapper.

◑ Glycerin suppositories often produce results within fifteen minutes to one hour. Be sure to consult your physician if you experience problems or do not get relief within a week.

Precautions

◑ Do not take any type of laxative if you have signs of appendicitis or inflamed bowel (e.g., stomach or lower abdominal pain, cramping, bloating, soreness, nausea, or vomiting). Check with your physician as soon as possible.

◑ Do not take any laxative for more than one week unless you have been told to do so by your physician. Many people tend to overuse laxatives, which often leads to dependence on the laxative action to produce a bowel movement. Discuss the use of laxatives with your health care professional in order to ensure that the laxative is used effectively as part of a comprehensive, healthy bowel management regimen.

◑ If you are pregnant, discuss with your physician the most appropriate type of laxative for you to use.

◑ Use only water to moisten the suppository prior to insertion in the rectum. Do not lubricate the suppository with mineral oil or petroleum jelly, which might affect the way the suppository works.

Possible Side Effects

➲ Side effects that may go away as your body adjusts to the medication and do not require medical attention unless they persist or are bothersome: skin irritation around the rectal area.

➲ Less common side effects that should be reported to your physician as soon as possible: rectal bleeding; blistering, or itching.

Chemical Name: Imipramine (im-**ip**-ra-meen)

Brand Name: Tofranil (U.S. and Canada)

Generic Available: Yes (U.S. and Canada)

Description: Imipramine is a tricyclic antidepressant used to treat mental depression. Its primary use in multiple sclerosis is to treat bladder symptoms, including urinary frequency and incontinence. Imipramine is also prescribed occasionally for the management of neurologic pain in MS.

Proper Usage

➲ To lessen stomach upset, take this medication with food, even for a daily bedtime dose, unless your physician has told you to take it on an empty stomach.

Precautions

➲ Imipramine adds to the effects of alcohol and other central nervous system depressants (e.g., antihistamines, sedatives, tranquilizers, prescription pain medications, seizure medications, muscle relaxants, sleeping medications), possibly causing drowsiness. Be sure that your physician knows if you are taking these or any other medications.

➲ This medication causes dryness of the mouth. Because continuing dryness of the mouth can increase the risk of dental disease, alert your dentist if you are taking imipramine.

➲ Imipramine may cause your skin to be more sensitive to sunlight than it is normally. Even brief exposure to sunlight may cause a skin rash, itching, redness or other discoloration of the skin, or severe sunburn. Stay out of the sun during the midday hours. Wear protective clothing and a sun block that has a skin protection factor (SPF) of at least 15.

➲ This medication may affect blood sugar levels of diabetic individuals. If you notice a change in the results of your blood or urine sugar tests, check with your physician.

➲ Do not stop taking imipramine without consulting your physician. The physician may want you to reduce the amount you are taking gradually in order to reduce the possibility of withdrawal symptoms such as headache, nausea, and/or an overall feeling of discomfort.

➲ Studies of imipramine have not been done in pregnant women. There have been reports of newborns suffering from muscle spasms and heart, breathing, and urinary problems when their mothers had taken tricyclic antidepressants immediately before delivery. Studies in animals have indicated the possibility of unwanted effects in the fetus.

◇ Imipramine passes into breast milk but has not been reported to have any effect on the nursing infant.

Possible Side Effects

⊃ Side effects that may go away as your body adjusts to the medication and do not require medical attention unless they continue for more than two weeks or are bothersome: dizziness; drowsiness*; headache; decreased sexual ability*; increased appetite; nausea; unusual tiredness or weakness*; unpleasant taste; diarrhea; heartburn; increased sweating; vomiting.

⊃ Uncommon side effects that should be reported to your physician as soon as possible: blurred vision*; confusion or delirium; constipation*; difficulty speaking or swallowing; eye pain*; fainting; fast or irregular heartbeat; hallucinations; loss of balance control*; nervousness or restlessness; problems urinating*; shakiness or trembling; stiffness of arms and legs*.

⊃ Rare side effects that should be reported to your physician as soon as possible: anxiety; breast enlargement in males and females; hair loss; inappropriate secretion of milk in females; increased sensitivity to sunlight; irritability; muscle twitching; red or brownish spots on the skin; buzzing or other unexplained sounds in the ears; skin rash; itching; sore throat and fever; swelling of face and tongue; weakness*; yellow skin.

⊃ Symptoms of acute overdose: confusion; convulsions; severe drowsiness*; enlarged pupils; unusual heartbeat; fever; hallucinations; restlessness and agitation; shortness of breath; unusual tiredness or weakness*; vomiting.

*Since it may be difficult to distinguish between certain common symptoms of MS and some side effects of imipramine, be sure to consult your health care professional if an abrupt change of this type occurs.

Chemical Name: Interferon beta-1a

Brand Name: Avonex (U.S.—approval in Canada is pending)

Generic Available: No

Description: Avonex is a medication manufactured by a biotechnological process from one of the naturally occurring interferons (a type of protein). It is made up of exactly the same amino acids (major components of proteins) as the natural interferon beta found in the human body. In a clinical trial of 380 ambulatory patients with relapsing-remitting MS, those taking the currently recommended dose of the medication had a reduced risk of disability progression, experienced fewer exacerbations, and showed a reduction in number and size of active lesions in the brain (as shown on MRI) when compared with the group taking a placebo.

Proper Usage

⊃ Avonex is given as a once-a-week intramuscular (IM) injection, usually in the large muscles of the thigh, upper arm, or hip. If your physician decides that you or a care partner can safely administer the injection, you will be taught how to reconstitute the medication (mix the sterile powder with the sterile water that is packaged with it) and instructed in safe and proper IM injection procedures. If you are unable to self-inject, and have no family member or friend available to do the injections, the injections will be given by your physician or nurse. Do not attempt to mix the medication or inject yourself until you are sure that you understand the procedures.

⊃ Avonex must be kept cold. Be sure to store it in a refrigerator both before and after the medication is mixed for injection. Do not expose the medication to high temperatures (in a glove compartment or on a window sill, for example) and do not allow it to freeze. Once the medication has been mixed for use, it is recommended that you administer the injection as soon as possible; the reconstituted powder should not be used once it has been stored in the refrigerator longer than six hours.

⊃ Do not reuse needles or syringes. Dispose of the syringes as directed by your physician and keep them out of the reach of children.

⊃ Since flu-like symptoms are a fairly common side effect during the initial weeks of treatment, it is recommended that the injection be given at bedtime. Taking acetaminophen (Tylenol®) or ibuprofen (Advil®) immediately prior to each injection and during the 24 hours following the injection will also help to relieve the flu-like symptoms.

Precautions

⊃ Avonex should not be used during pregnancy or by any woman who is trying to become pregnant. Women taking Avonex should use birth control measures at all times. If you want to become pregnant while being treated with Avonex, discuss the matter with your physician. If you become pregnant while using Avonex, stop the treatment and contact your physician.

⊃ There was no increase in depression reported by people receiving Avonex in the clinical trial. However, since depression and suicidal thoughts are known to occur with some frequency in MS, and depression and suicidal thoughts have been reported with high doses of various interferon products, it is recommended that individuals with a history of severe depressive disorder be closely monitored while taking Avonex.

⊃ Prior to starting treatment with Avonex, alert your physician if you have any prior history of a seizure disorder.

⊃ Prior to starting treatment with Avonex, alert your physician if you have any history of cardiac disease, including angina, congestive heart failure, or arrhythmia.

Possible Side Effects

⊃ Common side effects include flu-like symptoms (fatigue, chills, fever, muscle aches, and sweating). Most of these symptoms will tend to disappear after the initial few weeks of treatment. If they continue, become more severe, or cause you significant discomfort, be sure to talk them over with your physician.

⊃ Symptoms of depression, including ongoing sadness, anxiety, loss of interest in daily activities, irritability, low self-esteem, guilt, poor concentration, indecisiveness, confusion, and eating and sleep disturbances, should be reported promptly to your doctor.

Avonex Support Line: 800-456-2255

Chemical Name: Interferon beta-1b

Brand Name: Betaseron (U.S. and Canada)

Generic Available: No

Description: Betaseron is a medication manufactured by a biotechnological process from one of the naturally occurring interferons (a type of protein). In a clinical trial of 372 ambulatory patients with relapsing-remitting MS, those taking the currently recommended dose of the medication experienced fewer exacerbations, a longer time between exacerbations, and exacerbations that were generally less severe than those of patients taking a lower dose of the medication or a placebo. Additionally, patients on interferon beta-1b had no increase in total lesion area, as shown on MRI, in contrast to the placebo group, which had a significant increase.

Proper Usage

⊃ Betaseron is injected subcutaneously (between the fat layer just under the skin and the muscles beneath) every other day. The physician or nurse will instruct you in the preparation of the medication for injection and the injection procedure itself, using a specially designed set of training materials. Do not attempt to inject yourself until you are sure that you understand the procedures.

⊃ Betaseron must be kept cold. Be sure to store it in a refrigerator before and after the medication is mixed for injection.

⊃ Do not reuse needles or syringes. Dispose of the syringes as directed by your physician and keep them out of the reach of children.

⊃ Since flu-like symptoms are a common side effect associated with at least the initial weeks of taking Betaseron, it is recommended that the medication be taken at bedtime. Taking acetaminophen (Tylenol®) or ibuprofen (Advil®) thirty minutes before each injection will also help to relieve the flu-like symptoms.

⊃ Because injection site reactions (swelling, redness, discoloration, or pain) are relatively common, it is recommended that the sites be rotated according to a schedule provided for you by your physician.

Precautions

⊃ Betaseron should not be used during pregnancy or by any woman who is trying to become pregnant. Women taking Betaseron should use birth control measures at all times.

⊃ During the clinical trial of interferon beta-1b, there were four suicide attempts and one completed suicide among those taking interferon beta-1b. Although there is no evidence that the suicide attempts were related to the medication itself, it is recommended that individuals with a history of severe depressive disorder be close-ly monitored while taking Betaseron.

Possible Side Effects

⊃ Common side effects include flu-like symptoms (fatigue, chills, fever, muscle aches, and sweating) and injection site reactions (swelling, redness, discoloration, and pain). Most of these symptoms tend to disappear over time. If they continue, become more severe, or cause significant discomfort, be sure to talk them over with your physician. Contact your physician if the injection sites become inflamed, hardened, or lumpy, and do not inject into any area that has become hardened or lumpy.

⊃ Depression, including suicide attempts, has been reported by patients taking Betaseron. Common symptoms of depression are sadness, anxiety, loss of interest in daily activities, irritability, low self-esteem, guilt, poor concentration, indecisiveness, confusion, and eating and sleep disturbances. If you experience any of these symptoms for longer than a day or two, contact your physician promptly.

Betaseron Customer Service: 800-788-1467

Chemical Name: Magnesium hydroxide (mag-**nee**-zhum hye-**drox**-ide)

Brand Name: Phillips' Milk of Magnesia (available in granule form in Canada, in wafer form in the U.S., and in powder or effervescent powder in the U.S. and Canada) is one of several brands of bulk-forming laxative that are available over-the-counter.

Generic Available: No

Description: Magnesium hydroxide is an over-the-counter hyperosmotic laxative of the saline type that encourages bowel movements by drawing water into the bowel from surrounding body tissue. Saline hyperosmotic laxatives (often called "salts") are used for rapid emptying of the lower intestine and bowel. They are not to be used for the long-term management of constipation.

Proper Usage

⊃ Laxatives are to be used to provide short-term relief only, unless otherwise directed by the nurse or physician who is helping you to manage your bowel symptoms. A regimen that includes a healthy diet containing roughage (whole grain breads and cereals, bran, fruit, and green, leafy vegetables), six to eight full glasses of liquids each day, and some form of daily exercise is most important in stimulating healthy bowel function.

⊃ If your physician has recommended this laxative for management of constipation, follow his or her recommendations for its use. If you are treating yourself for constipation, follow the directions on the package insert. Results are often obtained ninety minutes to three hours after taking a hyperosmotic laxative. Be sure to consult your physician if you experience problems or do not get relief within a week.

⊃ Each dose should be taken with eight ounces or more of cold water or fruit juice. A second glass of water or juice with each dose is often recommended to prevent dehydration. If concerns about loss of bladder control keep you from drinking this amount of water, talk it over with the nurse or physician who is helping you manage your bowel and bladder symptoms.

Precautions

⊃ Do not take any type of laxative if you have signs of appendicitis or inflamed bowel (e.g., stomach or lower abdominal pain, cramping, bloating, soreness, nausea, or vomiting). Check with your physician as soon as possible.

⊃ Do not take any laxative for more than one week unless you have been told to do so by your physician. Many people tend to overuse laxatives, which often leads to dependence on the laxative action to produce a bowel movement. Discuss the use of laxatives with your health care professional in order to ensure that the laxative is used effectively as part of a comprehensive, healthy bowel management regimen.

⊃ Do not take any laxative within two hours of taking another medication because the desired effectiveness of the other medication may be reduced.

⊃ Although laxatives are commonly used during pregnancy, some types are better than others. If you are pregnant, consult your physician about the best laxative for you to use.

⊃ Some laxatives pass into breast milk. Although it is unlikely to cause problems for a nursing infant, be sure to let your physician know if you are using a laxative and breast-feeding at the same time.

Possible Side Effects

⊃ Side effects that may go away as your body adjusts to the medication and do not require medical attention unless they continue or are bothersome: cramping; diarrhea; gas; increased thirst.

⊃ Unusual side effects that should be reported to your physician as soon as possible: confusion; dizziness; irregular heartbeat; muscle cramps, unusual tiredness or weakness*.

*Since it may be difficult to distinguish between MS-related fatigue and the tiredness that can result from a hyperosmotic laxative, be sure to consult your health care professional if an abrupt change of this type occurs.

Chemical Name: Meclizine (**mek**-li-zeen)

Brand Name: Antivert (U.S.); Bonamine (Canada)

Generic Available: Yes (U.S.)

Description: Meclizine is used to prevent and treat nausea, vomiting, and dizziness.

Precautions

⊃ This drug adds to the effects of alcohol and other central nervous system depressants (e.g., antihistamines, sedatives, tranquilizers, prescriptions pain medications, seizure medications, muscle relaxants, sleeping medications), possibly causing drowsiness. Be sure that your physician knows if you are taking these or any other medications.

⊃ Meclizine may cause dryness of the mouth. If dryness continues for more than two weeks, speak to your physician or dentist since continuing dryness of the mouth may increase the risk of dental disease.

⊃ This medication has not been shown to cause birth defects or other problems in humans. Studies in animals have shown that meclizine given in doses many times the usual human dose causes birth defects such as cleft palate.

⊃ Although meclizine passes into breast milk, it has not been reported to cause problems in nursing babies. However, since this medication tends to decrease bodily secretions, it is possible that the flow of breast milk may be reduced in some women.

Possible Side Effects

⊃ Side effects that typically go away as your body adjusts to the medication and do not require medical attention unless they continue for more than two weeks or are bothersome: drowsiness*; blurred vision*; constipation*; difficult or painful urination; dizziness; dryness of mouth, nose, and throat; fast heartbeat; headache; loss of appetite; nervousness or restlessness; trouble sleeping; skin rash; upset stomach.

*Since it may be difficult to distinguish between certain common symptoms of MS and some side effects of meclizine, be sure to consult your health care professional if an abrupt change of this type occurs.

Chemical Name: Methenamine (meth-**en**-a-meen)

Brand Name: Hiprex; Mandelamine (U.S.); Hip-Rex; Mandelamine (Canada)

Generic Available: No

Description: Methenamine is an anti-infective medication that is used to help prevent infections of the urinary tract. It is usually prescribed on a long-term basis for individuals with a history of repeated or chronic urinary tract infections.

Proper Usage

⊃ Before you start taking this medication, check your urine with phenaphthazine paper or another test to see if it is acidic. Your urine must be acidic (pH 5.5 or below) for this medicine to work properly. Consult your health care professional about possible changes in your diet if necessary to increase the acidity of your urine (e.g., avoiding citrus fruits and juices, milk and other dairy products, antacids; eating more protein and foods such as cranberries and cranberry juice with added vitamin C, prunes, or plums).

Precautions

⊃ The effects of methenamine in pregnancy have not been studied in either humans or animals. Individual case reports have not shown that this medication causes birth defects or other problems in humans.

⊃ Methenamine passes into breast milk but has not been reported to cause problems in nursing infants.

Possible Side Effects

⊃ Side effects that typically go away as your body adjusts to the medication and do not require medical attention unless they continue or are bothersome: nausea; vomiting.

⊃ Unusual side effects that should be reported immediately to your physician: skin rash.

*Since it may be difficult to distinguish between certain common symptoms of MS and some side effects of methenamine, be sure to consult your health care professional if an abrupt change of this type occurs.

Chemical Name: Methylprednisolone (meth-ill-pred-**niss**-oh-lone)

Brand Name: Depo-Medrol (U.S. and Canada)

Generic Available: Yes (U.S. and Canada)

Description: Methylprednisolone is one of a group of corticosteroids (cortisone-like medications) that are used to relieve inflammation in different parts of the body. Corticosteroids are used in MS for the management of acute exacerbations because they have the capacity to close the damaged blood-brain barrier and reduce inflammation in the central nervous system. Although methylprednisolone is among the most commonly used corticosteroids in MS, it is only one of several possibilities. Other commonly used corticosteroids include dexamethazone, prednisone, betamethasone, and prednisolone. The following information pertains to all of the various corticosteroids.

Proper Usage

⊃ Most neurologists treating MS believe that high-dose corticosteroids given intravenously are the most effective treatment for an exacerbation, although the exact protocol for the drug's use may differ somewhat from one treating physician to another. Patients generally receive a four-day course of treatment (either in the hospital or as an outpatient), with doses of the medication spread throughout the day. This high-dose, intravenous steroid treatment is then typically followed by a gradually tapering dose of an oral corticosteroid (see Prednisone).

Precautions

⊃ Since corticosteroids can stimulate the appetite and increase water retention, it is advisable to follow a low-salt and/or potassium-rich diet and watch your caloric intake. Your physician will make specific dietary recommendations for you.

⊃ Corticosteroids can lower your resistance to infection and make any infection that you get more difficult to treat. Contact your physician if you notice any sign of infection, such as sore throat, fever, coughing, or sneezing.

⊃ Avoid close contact with anyone who has chicken pox or measles. Tell your physician right away if you think you have been exposed to either of these illnesses. Do not have any immunizations after you stop taking this medication until you have consulted your physician. People living in your home should not have the oral polio vaccine while you are being treated with corticosteroids since they might pass the polio virus on to you.

⊃ Corticosteroids may affect the blood sugar levels of diabetic patients. If you notice a change in your blood or urine sugar tests, be sure to speak to your physician.

⊃ The risk of birth defects for women taking corticosteroids is not known. Overuse of corticosteroids during pregnancy may slow the growth of the infant after birth. Animal studies have demonstrated that corticosteroids cause birth defects.

⊃ Corticosteroids pass into breast milk and may slow the infant's growth. If you are nursing or plan to nurse, be sure to discuss this with your physician. It may be necessary for you to stop nursing while taking this medication.

⊃ Corticosteroids may produce mood changes and/or mood swings of varying intensity. These mood alterations can vary from relatively mild to extremely intense, and can vary in a single individual from one course of treatment to another. Neither the patient nor the physician can predict with any certainty whether the corticosteroids are likely to precipitate these mood alterations. If you have a history of mood disorders (depression or bipolar disorder, for example), be sure to share this information with your physician. If you begin to experience mood changes or swings that feel unmanageable, contact your physician so that a decision can be made about whether or not you need an additional medication to help you until the mood alterations subside.

Possible Side Effects

⊃ Side effects that may go away as your body adjusts to the medication and do not require medical attention unless they continue or are bothersome: increased appetite; indigestion; nervousness or restlessness; trouble sleeping; headache; increased sweating; unusual increase in hair growth on body or face.

⊃ Less common side effects that should be reported as soon as possible to your physician: severe mood changes or mood swings; decreased or blurred vision*; frequent urination*.

⊃ Additional side effects that can result from the prolonged use of corticosteroids and should be reported to your physician: acne or other skin problems; swelling of the face; swelling of the feet or lower legs; rapid weight gain; pain in the hips or other joints (caused by bone cell degeneration); bloody or black, tarry stools; elevated blood pressure; markedly increased thirst (with increased urination indicative of diabetes mellitus); menstrual irregularities; unusual bruising of the skin; thin, shiny skin; hair loss; muscle cramps or pain. Once you stop this medication after taking it for a long period of time, it may take several months for your body to readjust.

*Since it may be difficult to distinguish between certain common symptoms of MS and some side effects of methylprednisolone, be sure to consult your health care professional if an abrupt change of this type occurs.

Chemical Name: Mineral oil

Mineral oil is available in a variety of brands in the U.S. and Canada.

Generic Available: Yes

Description: Mineral oil is a lubricant laxative that is taken by mouth. It encourages bowel movements by coating the bowel and the stool with a waterproof film that helps to retain moisture in the stool.

Proper Usage

⊃ Laxatives are to be used to provide short-term relief only, unless otherwise directed by the nurse or physician who is helping you to manage your bowel symptoms. A regimen that includes a healthy diet containing roughage (whole grain breads and cereals, bran, fruit, and green, leafy vegetables), six to eight full glasses of liquids each day, and some form of daily exercise is most important in stimulating healthy bowel function.

⊃ If your physician has recommended this type of laxative for management of constipation, follow his or her recommendations for its use. If you are treating yourself for constipation, follow the directions on the package insert. Mineral oil is usually taken at bedtime because it takes six to eight hours to produce results. Be sure to consult your physician if you experience problems or do not get relief within a week.

⊃ Mineral oil should not be taken within two hours of mealtime because the mineral oil may interfere with food digestion and the absorption of important nutrients.

⊃ Mineral oil should not be taken within two hours of taking a stool softener (see Docusate) because the stool softener may increase the amount of mineral oil that is absorbed by the body.

Precautions

⊃ Do not take any type of laxative if you have signs of appendicitis or inflamed bowel (e.g., stomach or lower abdominal pain, cramping, bloating, soreness, nausea, or vomiting). Check with your physician as soon as possible.

⊃ Do not take any laxative for more than one week unless you have been told to do so by your physician. Many people tend to overuse laxative products, which often leads to dependence on the laxative action to produce a bowel movement. Discuss the use of laxatives with your health care professional in order to ensure that the laxative is used effectively as part of a comprehensive, healthy bowel management regimen.

➲ Mineral oil should not be used very often or for long periods of time. Its gradual build-up in body tissues can cause problems, and may interfere with the body's absorption of important nutrients and vitamins A, D, E, and K.

➲ Do not take any laxative within two hours of taking another medication because the desired effectiveness of the other medication may be reduced.

➲ Mineral oil should not be used during pregnancy because it may interfere with absorption of nutrients in the mother and, if used for prolonged periods, cause severe bleeding in the newborn infant.

➲ Be sure to let your physician know if you are using a laxative and breast-feeding at the same time.

Possible Side Effects

➲ Uncommon side effect that usually does not need medical attention: skin irritation around the rectal area.

Chemical Name: Nitrofurantoin (nye-troe-fyoor-**an**-toyn)

Brand Name: Macrodantin (U.S. and Canada)

Generic Available: No

Description: Nitrofurantoin is an anti-infective that is used primarily to treat urinary tract infections.

Proper Usage

Nitrofurantoin should be taken with food or milk to lessen stomach upset and to promote your body's absorption of the medication.

➲ Finish the full course of treatment prescribed by your doctor, and avoid missing doses. Even if your symptoms disappear after a few days, stopping this medication prematurely may result in a return of the symptoms.

➲ If you miss a dose of this medication, take it as soon as possible, If, however, it is almost time for your next dose, skip the missed dose and go back to your regular dosing schedule. Do not double dose.

➲ The use of nitrofurantoin may cause your urine to become rusty-yellow or brownish. This change does not require medical treatment and does not need to be reported to your physician.

Precautions

➲ Nitrofurantoin can interact with, or alter the action of, a variety of other medications you may be taking. It is very important to let your physician know about all the medications you are taking so that necessary substitutions or dosage adjustments can be made.

➲ If you will be taking this medication over an extended period of time, your doctor will need to check your progress at regular visits. If your symptoms do not improve within a few days, or become worse, consult your physician.

➲ Individuals with diabetes may find that this medication alters the results of some urine sugar tests. Consult with your physician before changing your diet or the dose of your diabetes medicine.

➲ Certain medical conditions can affect the use of nitrofurantoin. Be sure to alert your physician about any medical conditions you have, especially glucose-6-phosphate dehydrogenase (G6PD) deficiency, kidney disease, or lung disease.

➲ Because nitrofurantoin can cause problems in infants, it should not be used by a woman who is within a week or two of her delivery date, or during labor and delivery.

⊃ Nitrofurantoin passes into breast milk in small amounts and may cause problems in nursing babies [especially those with glucose-6-phosphate dehydrogenase (G6PD) deficiency].

Possible Side Effects

⊃ Side effects that may go away as your body adjusts to the medication and do not require medical attention unless they continue or are bothersome: abdominal or stomach pain; diarrhea, loss of appetite, nausea, or vomiting. Rare side effects that should be reported to your doctor immediately: chest pain; chills; cough; fever; trouble breathing; dizziness; headache; numbness, tingling, or burning of face or mouth; unusual weakness or tiredness; itching; joint pain; skin rash; yellow eyes or skin.

⊃ Chronic use of this medication increases the body's need for vitamin B6 (pyridoxine) and supplements up to 25 mg are advised.

⊃ Chronic use of any antibiotic increases the risk of infection with resistant organisms.

Chemical Name: Nortriptyline(nor-**trip**-ti-leen)

Brand Name: Pamelor (U.S.); Aventyl (Canada)

Generic Available: Yes (U.S.)

Description: Nortriptyline is a tricyclic antidepressant used to treat mental depression. In multiple sclerosis, it is frequently used to treat painful paresthesias in the arms and legs (e.g., bands, burning sensations, pins and needles, stabbing pains) caused by damage to the pain-regulating pathways of the brain and spinal cord. Note: Other tricyclic antidepressants are also used for the management of neurologic pain symptoms: amitriptyline (Elavil—U.S. and Canada), clomipramine (Anafranil—U.S. and Canada), desipramine (Norpramin—U.S. and Canada), doxepin (Sinequan—U.S. and Canada), trimipramine (U.S. and Canada). While each of these medications is given in different doses, the precautions and side effects listed here for nortriptyline apply to these other tricyclic medications as well.

Precautions

⊃ Nortriptyline will add to the effects of alcohol and other central nervous system depressants (e.g., antihistamines, sedatives, tranquilizers, prescription pain medications, seizure medications, muscle relaxants, sleeping medications), possibly causing drowsiness. Be sure that your physician knows if you are taking these or any other medications.

⊃ This medication causes dryness of the mouth. Because continuing dryness of the mouth may increase the risk of dental disease, alert your dentist that you are taking nortriptyline.

⊃ This medication may cause your skin to be more sensitive to sunlight than it is normally. Even brief exposure to sunlight may cause a skin rash, itching, redness or other discoloration of the skin, or severe sunburn.

⊃ This medication may affect blood sugar levels of diabetic individuals. If you notice a change in the results of your blood or urine sugar tests, check with your doctor.

⊃ Do not stop taking this medication without consulting your doctor. The doctor may want you to reduce the amount you are taking gradually in order to reduce the possibility of withdrawal symptoms such as headache, nausea, and/or an overall feeling of discomfort.

⊃ Studies or nortriptyline have not been done in pregnant women. However, there have been reports of newborns suffering from muscle spasms and heart, breathing, and urinary problems when their mothers had taken tricyclic antidepressants immediately before delivery. Studies in animals have indicated the possibility of unwanted effects in the fetus.

⊃ Tricyclics pass into breast milk. Only doxepin (Sinequan) has been reported to cause drowsiness in the nursing baby.

Possible Side Effects

⊃ Side effects that may go away as your body adjusts to the medication and do not require medical attention unless they continue for more than two weeks or are bothersome: dryness of mouth; constipation; *increased appetite and weight gain;* dizziness; drowsiness; decreased sexual ability; headache; nausea; unusual tiredness or weakness; unpleasant taste; diarrhea; heartburn; increased sweating; vomiting.

⊃ Uncommon side effects that should be reported to the doctor as soon as possible: blurred vision; confusion or delirium; difficulty speaking or swallowing; eye pain; fainting; hallucinations; loss of balance control; nervousness or restlessness; problems urinating; shakiness or trembling; stiffness of arms and legs.

⊃ Rare side effects that should be reported to the doctor as soon as possible: anxiety; breast enlargement in males and females; increased sensitivity to sunlight; irritability; muscle twitching; red or brownish spots on the skin; buzzing or other unexplained sounds in the ears; skin rash; itching; sore throat and fever; swelling of face and tongue; weakness; yellow skin.

⊃ Symptoms of acute overdose: confusion; convulsions; severe drowsiness; enlarged pupils; unusual heartbeat; fever; hallucinations; restlessness and agitation; shortness of breath; unusual tiredness or weakness; vomiting.

*Since it may be difficult to distinguish between certain common symptoms of MS and some side effects of nortriptyline, be sure to consult your health care professional if an abrupt change of this type occurs.

Chemical Name: Oxybutynin (ox-i-**byoo**-ti-nin)

Brand Name: Ditropan (U.S. and Canada)

Generic Available: Yes (U.S.)

Description: Oxybutynin is an antispasmodic that helps decrease muscle spasms of the bladder and the frequent urge to urinate caused by these spasms.

Proper Usage

⮊ This medication is usually taken with water on an empty stomach, but your physician may want you to take it with food or milk to lessen stomach upset.

Precautions

⮊ This medication adds to the effects of alcohol and other central nervous system depressants (such as antihistamines, sedatives, tranquilizers, prescription pain medications, seizure medications, muscle relaxants). Be sure that your physician knows if you are taking these or any other medications.

⮊ This medication may cause your eyes to become more sensitive to light.

⮊ Oxybutynin may cause drying of the mouth. Since continuing dryness of the mouth can increase the risk of dental disease, alert your dentist if you are taking oxybutynin.

⮊ Oxybutynin has not been studied in pregnant women. It has not been shown to cause birth defects or other problems in animal studies.

⮊ This medication has not been reported to cause problems in nursing babies. However, since it tends to decrease body secretions, oxybutynin may reduce the flow of breast milk.

Possible Side Effects

⮊ Side effects that typically go away as your body adjusts to the medication and do not require medical attention unless they continue for a few weeks or are bothersome: constipation*; decreased sweating; unusual drowsiness*; dryness of mouth, nose, throat; blurred vision*; decreased flow of breast milk; decreased sexual ability*; difficulty swallowing*; headache; increased light sensitivity; nausea or vomiting; trouble sleeping; unusual tiredness or weakness*.

⮊ Less common side effects that should be reported to your physician immediately: difficulty in urination*.

*Since it may be difficult to distinguish between certain common symptoms of MS and some side effects of oxybutynin, be sure to consult your health care professional if an abrupt change of this type occurs.

Chemical Name: Papaverine (pa-**pav**-er-een)

Brand Name: None

Generic Available: Yes (U.S. and Canada)

Description: Papaverine belongs to a group of medicines called vasodilators, which cause blood vessels to expand, thereby increasing blood flow. Papaverine is used in MS to treat erectile dysfunction. When papaverine is injected into the penis, it produces an erection by increasing blood flow to the penis.

Proper Usage

➲ Papaverine should never be used as a sexual aid by men who are not impotent. If improperly used, this medication can cause permanent damage to the penis.

➲ Papaverine is available by prescription and should be used only as directed by your physician, who will instruct you in the proper way to give yourself an injection so that it is simple and essentially pain-free.

Precautions

➲ Do not use more of this medication or use it more often than it has been prescribed for you. Using too much of this medicine will result in a condition called priapism, in which the erection lasts too long and does not resolve when it should. Permanent damage to the penis can occur if blood flow to the penis is cut off for too long a period of time.

➲ Examine your penis regularly for possible lumps near the injection sites or for curvature of the penis. These may be signs that unwanted tissue is growing (called fibrosis), which should be examined by your physician.

Possible Side Effects

➲ Side effects that you should report to your physician so that he or she can adjust the dosage or change the medication: bruising at the injection site; mild burning along the penis; difficulty ejaculating; swelling at the injection site.

➲ Rare side effects that require immediate treatment: erection continuing for more than four hours. If you cannot be seen immediately by your physician, you should go to the emergency room for prompt treatment.

Chemical Name: Paroxetine (pa-**rox**-uh-teen)

Brand Name: Paxil (U.S. and Canada)

Generic Available: No

Description: Paroxetine is used to treat mental depression.

Proper Usage

⊃ Paroxetine may be taken with or without food, on an empty or full stomach.

Precautions

⊃ It may take up to four weeks or longer for you to feel the beneficial effects of this medication.

⊃ Your physician should monitor your progress at regularly scheduled visits in order to adjust the dose and help reduce any side effects.

⊃ This medication could add to the effects of alcohol and other central nervous system depressants (e.g., antihistamines, sedatives, tranquilizers, sleeping medicine, prescription pain medicine, barbiturates, seizure medication, muscle relaxants). Be sure that your physician knows if you are taking these or any other medications.

⊃ Paroxetine may cause dryness of the mouth. If your mouth continues to feel dry for more than two weeks, check with your physician or dentist. Continuing dryness of the mouth may increase the risk of dental disease.

⊃ This medication may cause you to become drowsy.

⊃ Studies have not been done in pregnant women. Studies in animals have shown that paroxetine may cause miscarriages and decreased survival rates when given in doses that are many times higher than the human dose.

⊃ Paroxetine passes into breast milk but has not been shown to cause any problems in nursing infants.

Possible Side Effects

⊃ Side effects that typically go away as your body adjusts to the medication and do not require medical attention unless they continue for several weeks or are bothersome: decrease in sexual drive or ability*; headache; nausea; problems urinating*; decreased or increased appetite; unusual tiredness or weakness*; tremor*; trouble sleeping; anxiety; agitation; nervousness or restlessness; changes in vision, including blurred vision*; fast or irregular heartbeat; tingling, burning, or prickly sensations*; vomiting.

➲ Unusual side effects that should be discussed with your physician as soon as possible: agitation; lightheadedness or fainting; muscle pain or weakness; skin rash; mood or behavior changes.

*Since it may be difficult to distinguish between certain common symptoms of MS and some side effects of paroxetine, be sure to consult your health care professional if an abrupt change of this type occurs.

Chemical Name: Pemoline (**pem**-oh-leen)

Brand Name: Cylert (U.S. and Canada)

Generic Available: No

Description: Pemoline is a mild central nervous system stimulant that has been used primarily to treat children with attention deficit hyperactivity disorder and adults with narcolepsy. It is used in multiple sclerosis to relieve certain types of fatigue.

Proper Usage

⊃ The usual starting dose for the treatment of fatigue in MS is 18.75 mg each morning for one week. If necessary, in order to manage the fatigue, the dosage can be gradually increased in increments of 18.75 mg and spread out over the early part of the day. In order to maximize the medication's effectiveness and minimize sleep disturbance, it should all be taken before mid-afternoon. The maximum dose of this medication is not known. Some individuals feel jittery or uncomfortable taking more than the minimum dose; others tolerate higher doses without discomfort. Typically, the drug is not prescribed at levels over 100–140 mgs per day for MS-related fatigue.

Precautions

⊃ Pemoline can increase hypertension. It should not be taken if you have angina and/or known coronary artery disease.

⊃ If you are taking pemoline in large doses for a long time, do not stop taking it without consulting your physician. Your physician may want you to reduce the amount you are taking gradually.

⊃ This drug may interact with the effects of alcohol and other central nervous system depressants (e.g., antihistamines, sedatives, tranquilizers, prescription pain medications, seizure medications, muscle relaxants, sleeping medications). Be sure your physician knows if you are taking these or any other medications.

⊃ Pemoline may cause some people to become dizzy or less alert than they are normally.

⊃ If you have been using this medicine for a long time and think you may have become mentally or physically dependent on it, check with your physician. Some signs of dependence on pemoline are a strong desire or need to continue taking the medicine; a need to increase the dose to receive the effects of the medicine; withdrawal side effects such as mental depression, unusual behavior, unusual tiredness* or weakness* after the medication is stopped.

⊃ Pemoline has not been shown to cause birth defects or other problems in humans. Studies in animals given large doses of pemoline have shown that it causes an increase in stillbirths and decreased survival of the offspring.

⊃ It is not known if pemoline is excreted in breast milk.

Possible Side Effects

Side effects of this medication have not been studied in adults. Side effects that have been reported by some adults in clinical practice include insomnia; elevated heart rate; nervousness; agitation; loss of appetite and weight loss; gastrointestinal upset, including constipation and diarrhea; hallucinations.

*Since it may be difficult to distinguish between certain common symptoms of MS and some side effects of pemoline, be sure to consult your health care professional if an abrupt change of this type occurs.

Chemical Name: Phenazopyridine (fen-az-oh-**peer**-i-deen)

Brand Name: Pyridium (U.S. and Canada)

Generic Available: Yes (U.S.)

Description: Phenazopyridine is used to relieve the pain, burning, and discomfort caused by urinary tract infections. It is not an antibiotic and will not cure the infection itself. This medication is available in the U.S. only with a prescription; it is available in Canada without a prescription. The medication comes in tablet form.

Precautions

⊃ The medication causes the urine to turn reddish orange. This effect is harmless and goes away after you stop taking phenazopyridine.

⊃ It is best not to wear soft contact lenses while taking this medication; phenazopyridine may cause permanent discoloration or staining of soft lenses.

⊃ Check with your physician if symptoms such as bloody urine, difficult or painful urination, frequent urge to urinate, or sudden decrease in the amount of urine appear or become worse while you are taking this medication.

⊃ Phenazopyridine has not been studied in pregnant women. It has not been shown to cause birth defects in animal studies.

⊃ It is not known whether this medication passes into breast milk. It has not been reported to cause problems in nursing babies.

Possible Side Effects

⊃ Uncommon side effects that typically go away as your body adjusts to the medication and do not require medical attention unless they continue or are bothersome: dizziness; headache; indigestion; stomach cramps or pain.

⊃ Unusual side effects that should be reported to your physician: blue or blue-purple color of skin; fever and confusion; shortness of breath; skin rash; sudden decrease in amount of urine; swelling of face, fingers, feet and/or lower legs; unusual weakness or tiredness*; weight gain; yellow eyes or skin.

*Since it may be difficult to distinguish between certain common symptoms of MS and some side effects of phenazopyridine, be sure to consult your health care professional if an abrupt change of this type occurs.

Chemical Name: Phenytoin (**fen**-i-toyn)

Brand Name: Dilantin (U.S. and Canada)

Generic Available: Yes (U.S.)

Description: Phenytoin is one of a group of hydantoin anticonvulsants that are used most commonly in the management of seizures in epilepsy. It is used in MS to manage painful dysesthesias (most commonly trigeminal neuralgia) caused by abnormalities in the sensory pathways in the brain and spinal cord.

Precautions

⊃ This drug may interact with the effects of alcohol and other central nervous system depressants (e.g., antihistamines, sedatives, tranquilizers, certain prescription pain medications, seizure medications, muscle relaxants, sleeping medications). Be sure your physician knows if you are taking these or any other medications.

⊃ Oral contraceptives (birth control pills) that contain estrogen may not be as effective if taken in conjunction with phenytoin. Consult with your physician about using a different or additional form of birth control to avoid unplanned pregnancies.

⊃ This medication may affect the blood sugar levels of diabetic individuals. Check with your physician if you notice any change in the results of your blood or urine sugar level tests while taking phenytoin.

⊃ Antacids or medicines for diarrhea can reduce the effectiveness of phenytoin. Do not take any of these medications within two to three hours of the phenytoin.

⊃ Before having any type of dental treatment or surgery, be sure to inform your physician or dentist if you are taking phenytoin. Medications commonly used during surgical and dental treatments can increase the side effects of phenytoin.

⊃ There have been reports of increased birth defects when hydantoin anticonvulsants were used for seizure control during pregnancy. It is not definitely known whether these medications were the cause of the problem. Be sure to tell your physician if you are pregnant or considering becoming pregnant.

⊃ Phenytoin passes into breast milk in small amounts.

Possible Side Effects

⊃ Side effects that may go away as your body adjusts to the medication and do not require medical attention unless they continue or are bothersome: constipation*; mild dizziness*; mild drowsiness*.

⊃ Side effects that should be reported to your physician: bleeding or enlarged gums; confusion; enlarged glands in the neck or underarms; mood or mental changes*; muscle weakness or pain*; skin rash or itching; slurred speech or stuttering; trembling; unusual nervousness or irritability.

⊃ Symptoms of overdose that require immediate attention: sudden blurred or double vision*; sudden severe clumsiness or unsteadiness*; sudden severe dizziness or drowsiness*; staggering walk*; severe confusion or disorientation.

*Since it may be difficult to distinguish between certain common symptoms of MS and some side effects of phenytoin, be sure to consult your health care professional if an abrupt change of this type occurs.

Chemical Name: Prednisone (**pred**-ni-sone)

Brand Name: Deltasone (U.S. and Canada)

Generic Available: Yes (U.S. and Canada)

Description: Prednisone is one of a group of corticosteroids (cortisone-like medicines) that are used to relieve inflammation in different parts of the body. Corticosteroids are used in MS for the management of acute exacerbations because they have the capacity to close the damaged blood-brain barrier and reduce inflammation in the central nervous system. Although prednisone is among the most commonly used corticosteroids in MS, it is only one of several different possibilities. Other commonly used corticosteroids include dexamethasone; prednisone; betamethasone; and prednisolone. The following information pertains to all of the various corticosteroids.

Proper Usage

⊃ Most neurologists treating MS believe that high-dose corticosteroids given intravenously are the most effective treatment for an MS exacerbation, although the exact protocol for the drug's use may differ somewhat from one treating physician to another. Patients generally receive a four-day course of treatment (either in the hospital or as an out-patient), with doses of the medication spread throughout the day (see Methylprednisolone). The high-dose, intravenous dose is typically followed by a gradually tapering dose of an oral corticosteroid (usually ranging in length from ten days to five or six weeks). Prednisone is commonly used for this oral taper. Oral prednisone may also be used instead of the high-dose, intravenous treatment if the intravenous treatment is not desired or is medically contraindicated.

Precautions

⊃ This medication can cause indigestion and stomach discomfort. Always take it with a meal and/or a glass or milk. Your physician may prescribe an antacid for you to take with this medication.

⊃ Take this medication exactly as prescribed by your physician. Do not stop taking it abruptly; your physician will give you a schedule that gradually tapers the dose before you stop it completely.

⊃ Since corticosteroids can stimulate the appetite and increase water retention, it is advisable to follow a low-salt and/or a potassium-rich diet and watch your caloric intake.

⊃ Corticosteroids can lower your resistance to infection and make any infection that you get more difficult to treat. Contact your physician

if you notice any sign of infection, such as sore throat, fever, coughing, or sneezing.

⊃ Avoid close contact with anyone who has chicken pox or measles.
Tell your physician immediately if you think you have been exposed
to either of these illnesses. Do not have any immunizations after
you stop taking this medication until you have consulted your physician. People living in your home should not have the oral polio vaccine while you are being treated with corticosteroids since they
might pass the polio virus on to you.

⊃ Corticosteroids may affect the blood sugar levels of diabetic
patients. If you notice a change in your blood or urine sugar tests,
be sure to discuss it with your physician.

⊃ The risk of birth defects in women taking corticosteroids during
pregnancy has not been studied. Overuse of corticosteroids during
pregnancy may slow the growth of the infant after birth. Animal
studies have demonstrated that corticosteroids cause birth defects.

⊃ Corticosteroids pass into breast milk and may slow the infant's
growth. If you are nursing or plan to nurse, be sure to discuss this
with your physician. It may be necessary for you to stop nursing
while taking this medication.

⊃ Corticosteroids can produce mood changes and/or mood swings
of varying intensity. These mood alterations can vary from relatively mild to extremely intense, and can vary in a single individual from one course of treatment to another. Neither the patient
nor the physician can predict with any certainty whether the corticosteroids are likely to precipitate these mood alterations. If
you have a history of mood disorders (depression or bipolar disorder, for example), be sure to share this information with your
physician. If you begin to experience unmanageable mood
changes or swings while taking corticosteroids, contact your
physician so that a decision can be made whether or not you
need an additional medication to help you until the mood alterations subside.

Possible Side Effects

⊃ Side effects that may go away as your body adjusts to the medication
and do not require medical attention unless they continue or are
bothersome: increased appetite; indigestion; nervousness or restlessness; trouble sleeping; headache; increased sweating; unusual
increase in hair growth on body or face.

⊃ Less common side effects that should be reported as soon as possible to your physician: severe mood changes or mood swings;
decreased or blurred vision*; frequent urination*.

⊃ Additional side effects that can result from the prolonged use of corticosteroids and should be reported to your physician: acne or other skin problems; swelling of the face; swelling of the feet or lower legs; rapid weight gain; pain in the hips or other joints (caused by bone cell degeneration); bloody or black, tarry stools; elevated blood pressure; markedly increased thirst (with increased urination indicative of diabetes mellitus); menstrual irregularities; unusual bruising of the skin; thin, shiny skin; hair loss; muscle cramps or pain. Once you stop this medication after taking it for a long period of time, it may take several months for your body to readjust.

*Since it may be difficult to distinguish between certain common symptoms of MS and some side effects of corticosteroids, be sure to consult your health care professional if an abrupt change of this type occurs.

Chemical Name: Propantheline (proe-**pan**-the-leen) bromide

Brand Name: Pro-Banthine (U.S. and Canada)

Generic Available: Yes (U.S.)

Description: Pro-Pantheline is one of a group of antispasmodic/anti-cholinergic medications used to relieve cramps or spasms of the stomach, intestines, and bladder. Propantheline is used in the management of neurogenic bladder symptoms to control urination.

Proper Usage

⊃ Take this medicine thirty minutes to one hour before meals unless otherwise directed by your physician.

Precautions

⊃ Do not stop this medication abruptly. Stop gradually to avoid possible vomiting, sweating, and dizziness.

⊃ Anticholinergic medications such as propantheline can cause blurred vision and light sensitivity. Make sure you know how you react to this medication before driving.

⊃ Anticholinergic medications may cause dryness of the mouth. If your mouth continues to feel dry for more than two weeks, check with your dentist. Continuing dryness of the mouth may increase the chance of dental disease.

⊃ No studies of the effects of this drug in pregnancy have been done in either humans or animals.

⊃ Anticholinergic medications have not been reported to cause problems in nursing babies. The flow of breast milk may be reduced in some women.

⊃ Be sure that your physician knows if you are taking a tricyclic antidepressant or any other anticholinergic medication. Taking propantheline with any of these may increase the anticholinergic effects, resulting in urinary retention.

Possible Side Effects

⊃ Side effects that typically go away as your body adjusts to the medication and do not require medical attention unless they continue for several weeks or are bothersome: constipation*; decreased sweating; dryness of mouth, nose, and throat; bloated feeling; blurred vision*; difficulty swallowing.

⊃ Unusual side effects that require immediate medical attention: inability to urinate; confusion; dizziness*; eye pain*; skin rash or hives.

⊃ Symptoms of overdose that require immediate emergency attention: unusual blurred vision*; unusual clumsiness or unsteadiness*;
unusual dizziness; unusually severe drowsiness*; seizures; hallucinations; confusion; shortness of breath; unusual slurred speech*;
nervousness; unusual warmth, dryness, and flushing of skin.

*Since it may be difficult to distinguish between certain common symp-
toms of MS and some side effects of propantheline, be sure to consult your
health care professional if an abrupt change of this type occurs.

Chemical Name: Psyllium hydrophilic mucilloid (**sill**-i-yum hye-droe-**fill**-ik **myoo**-sill-oid)

Brand Name: Metamucil (available in granule form in Canada, in wafer form in the U.S., and in powder or effervescent powder in the U.S. and Canada) is one of several available brands of bulk-forming laxative.

Generic Available: No

Description: Psyllium hydrophilic mucilloid is a bulk-forming oral laxative. This type of laxative is not digested by the body; it absorbs liquids from the intestines and swells to form a soft, bulky stool. The bowel is then stimulated normally by the presence of the bulky stool.

Proper Usage

⊃ Laxatives are to be used to provide short-term relief only, unless otherwise directed by the nurse or physician who is helping you to manage your bowel symptoms. A regimen that includes a healthy diet containing roughage (whole grain breads and cereals, bran, fruit, and green, leafy vegetables), six to eight full glasses of liquids each day, and some form of daily exercise is most important in stimulating healthy bowel function.

⊃ If your physician has recommended this laxative for management of constipation, follow his or her recommendations for its use. If you are treating yourself for constipation, follow the directions on the package insert. Results are often obtained in twelve hours but may take as long as two or three days. Be sure to consult your physician if you experience problems or do not get relief within a week.

⊃ In order for this type of bulk-forming laxative to work effectively without causing intestinal blockage, it is advisable to drink six to eight glasses (eight ounces) of water each day. Each dose of the laxative should be taken with eight ounces of cold water or fruit juice. If concerns about loss of bladder control keep you from drinking this amount of water, discuss it with the nurse or physician who is helping you manage your bowel and bladder symptoms.

Precautions

⊃ Do not take any type of laxative if you have signs of appendicitis or inflamed bowel (e.g., stomach or lower abdominal pain, cramping, bloating, soreness, nausea, or vomiting). Check with your physician as soon as possible.

⊃ Do not take any laxative for more than one week unless you have been told to do so by your physician. Many people tend to overuse laxatives, which often leads to dependence on the laxative action to produce a bowel movement. Discuss the use of laxatives with your health care professional in order to ensure that the laxative is used effectively as part of a comprehensive, healthy bowel management regimen.

➲ Do not take any laxative within two hours of taking another medication because the desired effectiveness of the other medication may be reduced.

➲ Bulk-forming laxatives are commonly used during pregnancy. Some of them contain a large amount of sodium or sugars, which may have possible unwanted effects such as increasing blood pressure or causing fluid retention. Look for those that contain lower sodium and sugar.

➲ Some laxatives pass into breast milk. Although it is unlikely to cause problems for a nursing infant, be sure to let your physician know if you are using a laxative and breast-feeding at the same time.

Possible Side Effects:

➲ Check with your physician as soon as possible if you experience any of the following: difficulty breathing; intestinal blockage; skin rash or itching; swallowing difficulty (feelings of lump in the throat).

Chemical Name: Sertraline (**ser**-tra-leen)

Brand Name: Zoloft (U.S. and Canada)

Generic Available: No

Description: Sertraline is used to treat mental depression.

Proper Usage

This medication should always be taken at the same time in relation to meals and snacks to make sure that it is absorbed in the same way. Because sertraline may be given to different individuals at different times of the day, you and your physician should discuss what to do about any missed doses.

Precautions

⊃ It may take four to six weeks for you to feel the beneficial effects of this medication.

⊃ Your physician should monitor your progress at regularly scheduled visits in order to adjust the dose and help reduce any side effects.

⊃ This medication could add to the effects of alcohol and other central nervous system depressants (e.g., antihistamines, sedatives, tranquilizers, sleeping medicine, prescription pain medicine, barbiturates, seizure medication, muscle relaxants). Be sure that your physician knows if you are taking these or any other medications.

⊃ Sertraline may cause dryness of the mouth. If your mouth continues to feel dry for more than two weeks, check with your physician or dentist. Continuing dryness of the mouth may increase the risk of dental disease.

⊃ This medication may cause drowsiness.

⊃ Studies have not been done in pregnant women. Studies in animals have shown that sertraline may cause delayed development and decreased survival rates of offspring when given in doses many times the usual human dose.

⊃ It is not known if sertraline passes into breast milk.

Possible Side Effects

⊃ Side effects that typically go away as your body adjusts to the medication and do not require medical attention unless they continue for several weeks or are bothersome: decreased appetite or weight loss; decrease sexual drive or ability*; drowsiness*; dryness of mouth; headache; nausea; stomach or abdominal cramps; tiredness or weakness*; tremor*; trouble sleeping; anxiety; agitation; nervousness or restlessness; changes in vision including blurred vision*; constipation*; fast or irregular heartbeat; flushing of skin; increased appetite; vomiting.

➲ Unusual side effects that should be discussed with your physician as soon as possible: fast talking and excited feelings or actions that are out of control; fever; skin rash; hives; itching.

*Since it may be difficult to distinguish between certain common symptoms of MS and some side effects of sertraline, be sure to consult your health care professional if an abrupt change of this type occurs.

Chemical Name: Sildenafil (sil-**den**-a-fil)

Brand Name: Viagra (U.S.)

Generic Available: No

Description: Sildenafil belongs to a group of medicines that delay the action of enzymes called phosphodiesterases, which can interfere with erectile function. Sildenafil is used to treat men with erectile dysfunction because it helps to maintain an erection that is produced when the penis is stroked. Without physical stimulation of the penis, sildenafil will not work to cause an erection. Sildenafil was not developed for use in women. (There are anecdotal reports of its use in women.)

Proper Usage

⊃ Sildenafil begins to work approximately 30 minutes after it is taken. The medication continues to work for up to four hours, although the effect is usually less after two hours.

⊃ Sildenafil is available by prescription and should be used only as directed by your physician. The dose of this medication will be different for different patients. Do not take more of this medication than has been prescribed for you.

Precautions

⊃ Sildenafil can interact with, or interfere with the action of, other medications you may be taking. Be sure to inform your physician of all other medications you are taking so that appropriate substitutions or dosage adjustments can be made. Sildenafil should not be used by men who are using nitrates such as nitroglycerin (e.g., Nitrostat or Transderm-Nitro) to lower their blood pressure; sildenafil can cause the blood pressure to drop too far.

⊃ The presence of certain medical problems can interfere with the use of sildenafil. Be sure to inform your doctor if you have any of the following medical problems: an abnormality of the penis (including a curved penis or birth defect); bleeding problems; retinitis pigmentosa; any conditions causing thickened blood or slower blood flow (e.g., leukemia, multiple myeloma, polycythemia, sickle cell disease, or thrombocycemia); a history of priapism (erection lasting longer than six hours); heart or blood disease; severe kidney problems; severe liver problems.

⊃ Sildenafil has not been studied in combination with other medications that are used in the treatment of erectile dysfunction. At the present time, it is not recommended that these drugs be used together.

Possible Side Effects

➲ Side effects that you should report to your physician so that he or she can adjust the dose or change the medication: flushing; headache; nasal congestion; stomach discomfort after meals; diarrhea.

➲ Rare side effects that should be discussed with your physician: abnormal vision (e.g., blurred vision, seeing shades of colors differently than before, sensitivity to light); bladder pain; cloudy or bloody urine; dizziness; increased frequency of urination; painful urination. *Note:* There are a variety of other possible side effects that have not yet been definitely shown to be caused by sildenasfil. Therefore, if you notice any other effects that cause you concern, be sure to talk them over with your doctor.

Chemical Name: Sodium phosphate

Brand Name: Fleet Enema (U.S. and Canada)

Generic Available: No

Description: Sodium phosphate enemas are available over-the-counter.

Proper Usage

⊃ Rectal enemas are to be used to provide short-term relief only, unless otherwise directed by the nurse or physician who is helping you to manage your bowel symptoms. A regimen that includes a healthy diet containing roughage (whole grain breads and cereals, bran, fruit, and green, leafy vegetables), six to eight full glasses of liquids each day, and some form of daily exercise is most important in stimulating healthy bowel function.

⊃ If your physician has recommended this rectal laxative for management of constipation, follow his or her recommendations for its use. If you are treating yourself for constipation, follow the directions on the package insert.

⊃ Results usually occur within two to five minutes. Be sure to consult your physician if you notice rectal bleeding, blistering, pain, burning, itching, or other signs of irritation that was not present before you began using a sodium phosphate enema.

Precautions

⊃ Do not use any type of laxative if you have signs of appendicitis or inflamed bowel (e.g., stomach or lower abdominal pain, cramping, bloating, soreness, nausea, or vomiting). Check with your physician as soon as possible.

⊃ Do not use any laxative for more than one week unless you have been told to do so by your physician. Many people tend to overuse laxatives, which often leads to dependence on the laxative action to produce a bowel movement. Discuss the use of laxatives with your health care professional in order to ensure that the laxative is used effectively as part of a comprehensive, healthy bowel management regimen.

⊃ If you are pregnant, discuss with your physician the most appropriate type of laxative for you to use.

Possible Side Effects

⊃ Side effect that may go away as your body adjusts to the medication and does not require medical attention unless it persists or is bothersome: skin irritation in the rectal area.

➲ Unusual side effects that should be reported to your physician as soon as possible: rectal bleeding, blistering, burning, itching.

Chemical   Name: Sulfamethoxazole   (sul-fa-meth-**ox**-a-zole)   and
trimethoprim (try-**meth**-oh-prim) combination

Brand Name: Bactrim; Septra (U.S. and Canada)

Generic Available: Yes (U.S.)

Description: Sulfamethoxazole and trimethoprim combination is used in
multiple sclerosis to treat (and sometimes to prevent) urinary tract
infections.

Proper Usage

⊃ This medication is best taken with a full glass (eight ounces) of
water. Additional water should be taken each day to help prevent
unwanted effects.

⊃ Finish the full course of treatment prescribed by your physician.
Even if your symptoms disappear after a few days, stopping this
medication prematurely may result in a return of the symptoms.

⊃ This medication works most effectively when it is maintained at a
constant level in your blood or urine. To help keep the amount
constant, do not miss any doses. It is best to take the doses at evenly spaced times during the day and night. For maximum effectiveness, four doses per day would be spaced at six-hour intervals.

Precautions

⊃ This medication may cause dizziness.

⊃ If taken for a long time, sulfamethoxazole and trimethoprim combination may cause blood problems. It is very important that your
physician monitor your progress at regular visits.

⊃ This medication can cause changes in the blood, possibly resulting
in a greater chance of certain infections, slow healing, and bleeding of the gums. Be careful with the use of your toothbrush, dental
floss, and toothpicks. Delay dental work until your blood counts are
completely normal. Check with your dentist if you have questions
about oral hygiene during treatment.

⊃ This medication may cause your skin to become more sensitive to
sunlight. Stay out of direct sunlight during the midday hours, wear
protective clothing, and apply a sun block product that has a skin
protection factor (SPF) of at least 15.

⊃ Sulfamethoxazole and trimethoprim combination has not been
reported to cause birth defects or other problems in humans. Studies in mice, rats, and rabbits have shown that some sulfonamides
cause birth defects, including cleft palate and bone problems. Studies in rabbits have also shown that trimethoprim causes birth

defects, as well as a decrease in the number of successful pregnancies.

⊃ Sulfamethoxazole and trimethoprim pass into breast milk. This medication is not recommended for use during breast-feeding. It may cause liver problems, anemia, and other problems in nursing babies.

Possible Side Effects

⊃ Side effects that may go away as your body adjusts to the medication and do not require medical attention unless they continue or are bothersome: diarrhea; dizziness; headache; loss of appetite; nausea or vomiting.

⊃ Less common side effects that should be reported to your physician immediately: itching; skin rash; aching of muscles and joints; difficulty in swallowing; pale skin; redness, blistering, peeling, or loosening of skin; sore throat and fever; unusual bleeding or bruising; unusual tiredness or weakness*; yellow eyes or skin.

---

*Since it may be difficult to distinguish between the tiredness that is common in MS (especially in the presence of an infection) and this side effect of sulfamethoxazole and trimethoprim combination, be sure to consult your physician if an abrupt change of this type occurs.

Chemical Name: Tolterodine (tol-ter-o-dine)

Brand Name: Detrol (U.S.) (and Canada?)

Generic Available: No

Description: Tolterodine is an antispasmodic that is used to treat bladder spasms causing urinary frequency, urgency, or urge incontinence.

Proper Usage

⊃ Take only the amount of this medication that has been prescribed for you by your doctor; taking more than the prescribed amount can cause adverse effects.

⊃ If you miss a dose of this medication, take it as soon as possible. If, however, it is almost time for your next dose, skip the missed dose and go back to your regular schedule. Do not double dose.

Precautions

⊃ Individuals with any of the following medical problems should not take this medication: gastric retention, urinary retention, or narrow angle or uncontrolled glaucoma. Tolterodine can aggravate each of these conditions.

⊃ Tolterodine may cause dizziness or drowsiness; use caution when driving or doing any activities that require alertness.

⊃ Tolterodine may cause drying of the mouth. Since continued dryness of the mouth can increase the risk of dental disease, alert your dentist if you are taking this medication.

⊃ This medication has not been studied in pregnancy. However, it has been shown in animal studies to result in increased embryo deaths, reduced birth weight, and increased incidence of fetal abnormalities. If you are pregnant or planning to become pregnant, do not start this medication before you have discussed it with your physician.

⊃ It is not known whether tolterodine passes into breast milk. Since tolterodine is known to pass into the milk of nursing animals, causing temporary reduction in weight gain in the offspring, women should stop taking this drug as long as they are nursing.

Possible Side Effects

⊃ Comment: An excellent medicine for the spastic bladder with fewer side effects than most others. But, as do other antispastic medications, increases incomplete emptying.

⊃ Side effects that will typically go away as your body adjusts to the medication and do not require medical attention unless they continue for a few weeks or are bothersome: dry mouth; dizziness; headache; fatigue; gastrointestinal symptoms, including abdominal pain, constipation, or diarrhea; difficult urination.

⊃ Less common side effects that should be reported to your physician immediately: abnormal vision, including difficulty adjusting to distances; urinary tract infection.

Chemical Name: Venlafaxine (ven-la-**fax**-een)

Brand Name: Effexor (U.S. and Canada)

Generic Available: No

Description: Venlafaxine is used to treat mental depression.

Dosage and Proper Usage

⊃ Unless your physician has instructed otherwise, this medication should be taken with food or on a full stomach to reduce the chances of stomach upset.

⊃ If you miss a dose of this medication, take it as soon as possible. If, however, it is within two hours of your next dose, skip the missed dose and return to your regular schedule. Do not double dose.

Precautions

⊃ It may take four to six weeks for you to feel the beneficial effects of this medication.

⊃ Your physician should monitor your progress at regularly scheduled visits in order to adjust the dose and help reduce any side effects.

⊃ Do not stop taking this medication without consulting your physician. The doctor may want you to reduce the amount you are taking gradually in order to decrease unwanted side effects.

⊃ This medication could add to the effects of alcohol and other central nervous system depressants (e.g., antihistamines, sedatives, tranquilizers, sleeping medicine, prescription pain medication, barbiturates, seizure medication, muscle relaxants). Be sure that your doctor know if you are taking these or any other medications.

⊃ Venlafaxine may cause dryness of the mouth. If your mouth continues to feel dry for more than two weeks, check with your physician or dentist. Continuing dryness of the mouth may increase the risk of dental disease.

⊃ This medication may cause you to become drowsy or to have double vision.

⊃ Venlafaxine may cause dizziness, lightheadedness, or fainting, especially when you stand from a sitting or lying position. If rising slowly from a sitting or lying position does not relieve the problem, consult your physician.

⊃ Studies have not been done in pregnant women. However, studies in animals have shown that venlafaxine may cause decreased survival rates of offspring when given in doses that are many times the usual dose for humans. If you are pregnant, or planning to become pregnant, do not start this medication before you have discussed it with your physician.

⊃ It is not known whether venlafaxine passes into breast milk. Mothers who are taking this medication and wish to breast-feed should discuss this with their doctor.

Possible Side Effects

⊃ Side effects that will typically go away as your body adjusts to the medication and do not require medical attention unless they continue for several weeks or are bothersome: abnormal dreams; anxiety or nervousness; constipation; dizziness; drowsiness; dryness of mouth; tingling or burning sensations; decreased appetite; nausea; stomach or abdominal cramps; trouble sleeping; tiredness; tremor.

⊃ Unusual side effects that should be discussed with the doctor as soon as possible: changes in vision or double vision; changes in sexual desire or ability; headache; chest pain; fast heartbeat; itching or skin rash; mood or mental changes; uncontrolled excitability; high blood pressure.

⊃ Symptoms of overdose include: extreme drowsiness, tiredness, or weakness.

⊃ Efflexor is a new antidepressant with features of both SRUI and tricyclic antidepressants. It is frequently effective and well tolerated.

Index

3